The DASH Diet Weight Loss Blueprint

How to Lower Your Blood Pressure Naturally While Losing Inches off Your Waist

Elaine Summers

Absolute Life Publishing

WYOMING - USA

Elaine Summers
support@summernutrition.org

Ordering Information:
Quantity sales. Special discounts are available on quantity purchases by corporations, associations, and others. For details, contact the "Special Sales Department" at the address above.

The DASH Diet Weight Loss Blueprint/ Elaine Summers. —4th ed.
ISBN 978-1-7364109-5-0

Contents

Welcome to the DASH Diet 1

What is the DASH Diet? 7

Superstar Nutrients 13

Fabulous Food Groups of DASH 19

Implementing DASH 37

Custom Meal Plan 53

Supercharge Your Weight Loss 67

Staying on Track 75

Getting Nerdy with DASH 83

Blood Pressure & Hypertension 91

Shopping for DASH 103

Flex Your Culinary Muscles 111

Final Thoughts 119

Simply Delicious Recipes 129

CHAPTER ONE

Welcome to the DASH Diet

Welcome to your one-stop DASH diet guide! In this book, you will learn the ins and outs of the DASH diet with two primary goals in mind: lowering your blood pressure and losing weight.

You might have discovered this guide after being diagnosed with hypertension, or you are trying to improve your lifestyle to avoid such a diagnosis. Being diagnosed with high blood pressure or hypertension can lead to thoughts of dealing with debilitating health problems for the rest of your life, but understand that high blood pressure is a manageable condition and can be controlled with the right knowledge and a few lifestyle changes. You are already on the right track by picking up this book and preparing to take action to better your health, so we commend you for taking the first step!

Will DASH Work for You?

DASH is an acronym for Dietary Approaches to Stop Hypertension. Therefore, DASH was explicitly created to help those who suffer from high blood pressure, like yourself, to lower their blood pressure naturally.

If you have any doubts about whether or not DASH will work, rest assured knowing DASH is evidence-based, meaning many studies and research have been conducted to confirm the effectiveness of the DASH diet. Many times over, results have shown how DASH is effective in lowering blood pressure and improving other conditions such as cholesterol and blood sugar with just food alone, regardless of age, gender, socioeconomic status, and ethnicity. The studies will be reviewed in-depth later in this book.

DASH was not created with weight loss in mind but, as we will discuss in this guide, has shown that weight loss is achievable with a slight increase in physical activity and minor caloric reductions. We'll show you how the standard DASH diet can be tailored to promote healthy weight loss, while remaining true to everything that makes DASH so great. Additionally, we will go over techniques that will help you boost your weight loss efforts, beyond what the nutrition section already offers. All of this combined will give you the best possible chance to obtain your ideal weight.

DASH should work for you as much as you allow it, meaning it is up to you to follow the diet and maintain it to reap the maximum benefits it has to offer and to manage your blood pressure at a healthy range. There will be times when you may fall out of the diet, but don't let that stop you from following it. Go ahead and enjoy that chocolate cake at your birthday party but, afterward, remember to come back to DASH.

There are a few special circumstances that might affect how well DASH will work for you. The first is if you are currently under a lot of stress. In addition to severely affecting blood pressure, studies have shown that times of stress can make weight loss significantly harder to achieve.[1] Stressful events can be debilitating. If stress is causing you depression, anxiety, or severely affecting your mood, it's advised to work on managing your stress and seeking professional help. This will greatly increase your chances of reaching your desired weight and lowering your blood pressure.

The second situation that can play a role in how well DASH works for you, is whether you suffer from any type of eating disorder. We consider eating disorders to be very serious, whether over- or under-eating. While anyone who is overweight with an eating disorder can do well on this diet, it is recommended that if you feel you might suffer from an eating disorder, you seek professional counseling while following this guide. Recognizing these kinds of factors will help you identify areas in your life that can affect your blood pressure and weight loss journey.

Before jumping into the DASH diet, let's take a moment to understand your WHY. Why are you embarking on the DASH journey? Is it to lower your blood pressure enough to where you don't have to rely on medication anymore? Is it to lose some weight so you can move around more comfortably and have more energy to keep up with your friends and loved ones? What events made you want to lose weight and improve your blood pressure? Whether you were placed on blood pressure medication, or have been struggling with your weight for most of your life, write down your WHY on a note and place it in the front of this book so you can use those events as a motivator throughout your DASH journey.

What to Expect

The DASH diet will require a few lifestyle changes, but you are encouraged to integrate these changes slowly into your daily routine. We will start with dietary changes combined with cooking and food prep, and slowly dedicate more time to exercise. Following DASH will put you in the kitchen more often, which will help you control the amount of salt in your food. The more time you spend in the kitchen, the less time you spend dining out on foods high in sodium, saturated fats, cholesterol, trans fats, and added sugars.

In this book we will go into detail on cooking techniques that are healthy and DASH-approved, what basic cooking tools you need, how to prepare food safely for yourself and others, what kitchen staples you should have at all times, and how to plan your meals. To help you when you go grocery shopping, we will learn how to read nutrition labels and how to identify the amount of sodium in a package of food. We will also learn tips for eating out to help you stay within your goals for the DASH diet. The diet will be focused on preparing low-sodium meals, increasing your fruits and vegetables, and educating yourself on healthy proteins and whole-grain sources. All while eating foods you enjoy. For those who are vegetarian, DASH is also vegetarian-friendly!

In terms of exercise, we will look at increasing ways to move and setting realistic goals. Increasing and maintaining physical activity will help you not only lose weight but also lower your blood pressure. By lowering your blood pressure and losing weight through diet and exercise, expect a few positive changes in your life. Improving your health naturally boosts energy and improves sleep, which can typically have a positive impact on your productivity at work and energy in your personal life.

Your weight loss will also have a positive effect on your blood pressure. Less weight means less strain on your cardiovascular system, which can further lower your blood pressure. DASH does not promote rapid weight loss, but rather a slow and steady, sustainable weight loss. This is the ideal way to lose weight permanently. Losing weight too quickly signals your body that you are on a fast, which tells your body that food must be scarce.

Your body will then kick in its survival instincts to retain body fat and increase your appetite to regain any weight you lost. Thus, slow and easy is the best way to lose weight!

Before You Start

To see your progress and determine if the DASH diet and lifestyle changes are working for you and your goals, make an effort to log your blood pressure readings at least once a week by purchasing your own blood pressure monitor and cuff. There are a few tips and techniques to measure your blood pressure at home accurately.

As recommended by the American Heart Association,[2] refrain from exercising or drinking caffeine up to 30 minutes before you take your blood pressure readings. Sit straight with your feet flat on the ground, stay relaxed for 5 minutes, then take the reading. To ensure your measurement is accurate, take two or three readings one minute apart, and record all the readings. Every time you measure, try conducting it around the same time of day as well, such as every Friday at 8:00 am.

If you have high blood pressure, you probably heard the words systolic and diastolic to describe blood pressure readings. Let's say your last reading was 140/90 mm Hg. The top number, 140, is your systolic blood pressure, which represents the force of your heart when it contracts to pump blood. The bottom number, 90, is your diastolic blood pressure, which is the force of your heart when it is resting between beats. The unit of measurement to measure the strength of blood pressure is in mm Hg, short for millimeters of Mercury. The standard for normal blood pressure is 120/80 mm Hg or less.

We also recommend logging your food intake daily. You don't have to be specific with calories and the weight of your meals, simply write down what you are eating. You may discover you eat more snacks than you think or find that you eat enough fruits and vegetables but just need to lower your number of sodas. Comparing your food log against the prescribed DASH guidelines will give you a good indicator of areas you can work on in your diet to even start seeing results within the first week.

Antihypertensive Medication

If your doctor prescribed antihypertensive medication, take them as prescribed alongside the DASH diet for the time being.[3] Over time, you may lower your blood pressure enough to where your doctor can recommend that you stop the medication altogether.

During checkups, show your doctor your log of blood pressure readings. This will spark a conversation about potentially being taken off your medications if the DASH diet and physical activity start to lower your blood pressure. If you need extra support nutritionally, ask your doctor for a referral to an outpatient Registered Dietitian who can touch base with you regularly to help you reach your goals.

Are you ready? Let's get started!

CHAPTER TWO

What is the DASH Diet?

The American Diet and Its Effects

Before we start discussing what the DASH diet is, we will look into the facts and statistics of our nation's nutrition and health issues to gain a better understanding of why DASH was created. While reading the data may cause you to feel uneasy, it is relevant to understanding why we are facing such problems as hypertension and obesity. While genetics and environmental factors may play a role, there is a cause and effect when it comes to health. Once you understand the causes of hypertension, you can understand how to take action to better your blood pressure and lose weight. Best of all, you will be able to maintain it, so this doesn't become a burden on your life again.

Nutrition

As Americans, we are busy people. Working long hours, being stuck in traffic, and balancing our personal lives have created a problem in terms of time and energy. As a solution, our society has been built on ease and convenience. For example, you can get your coffee-to-go, pick up fast food in a drive-through, and heat frozen meals for dinner. Unfortunately, most of these options are high in saturated fats, sodium, refined carbohydrates, omega-6 fatty acids, and sugar.[4]

A recent survey found that 90% of Americans eat more than the recommended maximum of 2,300 mg of sodium (about 1 teaspoon of salt) a day.[5] Our average consumption of sodium is about 3,400 mg. If we can cut back at least 1,200 mg of sodium from what we usually eat, we can save over $20 billion in annual healthcare costs. The American diet also happens to be low in fruits and vegetables. In 2018, the Centers for Disease Control and Prevention reported that 12.2% of adults in the United States eat the daily recommended number of fruits, and only 9.3% meet the recommended vegetable intake.[6] That's only 1 in every 10 adults.

Eating enough fruits and vegetables provides your body with the essential micronutrients you need to prevent many diseases and can even protect you from chronic illnesses like diabetes, cancer, and heart diseases.[6] Fruits and veggies also contain potassium, magnesium, and calcium, which are micronutrients needed to maintain optimal blood pressure. Take a quick moment to remember how many fruits and vegetables you ate in the last couple of days. Should you be adding more? Later on, we will go over the daily amounts of fruits and vegetables recommended by the DASH diet and how to achieve it.

Why are we not eating enough of these essential foods? The answer may be as simple as access to produce, cost of fresh groceries,[6] gaps in nutrition knowledge, and lack of cooking skills. Many communities have recognized this problem and are working on solutions such as delivering meal kits and groceries, involving children in school gardens, adding salad bars in school cafeterias,[6] and having adults participate in nutrition education courses and exercise classes through worksite wellness programs. More food banks are becoming selective in the types of foods they distribute, ensuring their communities receive whole grains and produce rather than packaged snacks. There has also been an increase in farmers' markets with 2.7 farmers' markets for every 100,000 US citizens.[6]

Sedentary Lifestyle and Obesity

It's easy to be inactive, especially if your career requires you to work at a desk or behind the wheel. Gym memberships can be expensive, and the weather or neighborhood you live in may not be ideal for walking outside. What do your situation and space look like? When was the last time you went for a walk or had the urge to go for a walk? A rule of thumb for physical activity is to be moderately active for at least 30 minutes a day, but less than 5% of adults meet this number. And only one-third of adults meet the recommended minimum of 150 minutes physical activity per week.[5]

Pairing our physical inactivity with our current diet, we run into the issue of obesity in the United States. Overweightness and obesity are ongoing problems in our nation. It is a factor in the development of type 2 diabetes mellitus, hypertension, stroke, liver and gallbladder disease, sleep apnea, coronary heart disease, osteoarthritis, reproductive issues, and various cancers.[7]

Being overweight or obese makes it three times more prevalent for getting type 2 diabetes and two times more likely to have hypertension than individuals with a healthy body mass index.[7] Even more shocking is that it is projected that 50% of adults in the US will be obese by 2030.[5] Diseases related to obesity cost about $190 billion in the United States per year.[5] If we break this down to an individual person, being obese costs you $4,880 per year if you're a woman and $2,650 if you're a man.

Since 2016, 1 out of 3 American adults have high blood pressure[8] and, according to the World Health Organization, 1 billion people worldwide have hypertension. Furthermore, this chronic condition is responsible for 12.5% of deaths each year.[9] These statistics might seem morbid, but it is not all doom and gloom. All of this can be prevented with a little exercise, and a diet low in sodium and high in potassium,[10] such as DASH.

Enter the DASH Diet

With heart disease being the number one killer in the United States,[11] it was only a matter of time until a solution was created and trialed to help fight this growing issue. And so, DASH was born in the early 1990s by the National Institute of Health (NIH).[4]

DASH was initially created as a nutrition intervention to promote a healthy diet without considering sodium reduction or lifestyle changes such as tobacco cessation and increased physical activity. While you may find it odd that sodium reduction was not part of the initial trial, researchers initially only wanted to figure out if increasing fruits and vegetables alone will do the trick in lowering blood pressure. Once they found out that it worked, they then went into a second trial to test reduced sodium. DASH was also created in hopes to find an alternative to using medications to decrease blood pressure.[12]

The main premise of the DASH diet consists of eating fruits, vegetables, whole grains, beans, heart-healthy fats, nuts, seeds, lean meats, plant proteins, and low-fat dairy.[4] A positive side-effect of eating more of these types of foods, is your overall intake of fast food, sodas, added sugar, and sodium should decrease. All aiding in naturally improving your blood pressure. We will be going into great detail about the specific foods in DASH once we reach the nutrition section.

Know that the DASH diet is not a fad diet. It was designed to include all macronutrients and major micronutrients. The food choices for DASH are also broad enough where you can find the foods at your local grocery store that is both accessible and affordable. It can be used both as a treatment and as a prevention for hypertension.

Later in this guide, we will go into detail on five critical research trials conducted on DASH. They hold valuable information on the types of subjects chosen to participate, how well designed the experiments were to get accurate results but, most importantly, how DASH is an evidence-based diet which continues to get exceptional results in lowering blood pressure. Because the diet is safe, nutritious, and easy to follow, the DASH diet has even been ranked as the best overall diet by U.S. News and World Report for eight years in a row after comparing it to 40 other diets.[9]

Health Benefits of DASH

Although we have mentioned quite shocking statistics, don't let this discourage you. Use it as a tool and motivator to improve your health. Luckily, we are living in a time where research studies have proven that DASH can lower blood pressure. Diet is your first line of treatment for hypertension, but you can improve its effects by reducing alcohol intake, quitting smoking, and exercising regularly.[4] If you follow the DASH diet, you should see your blood pressure improve in less than two weeks.[9] While excessively lowering sodium is not required in the DASH diet, pairing it with very-low-sodium eating will yield even better results, especially if you have exceptionally high blood pressure.[9]

Weight loss should result naturally while on the DASH diet, especially if you follow the guidelines in this book. The amount of weight loss depends on several factors, such as calorie restriction and exercise,[4] but a 5 to 10% weight loss in the first six months is what we aim for. A few extra health benefits from weight loss may include better management of Type 2 diabetes mellitus, reduced risk of stroke and other cardiovascular events, lowered cholesterol, triglycerides, and blood glucose, and less risk of colon cancer.[4]

On the flip side, there are no known side effects of DASH. Based on research, it is a healthy and sustainable diet with enough flexibility to prevent you from breaking your diet. DASH has become one of the national guidelines for healthy eating. Any health benefits you gain from being on the diet, such as lower blood pressure and weight loss, can be maintained as long as you can continue DASH.

What brought you here?

Each of us has a different journey that brought us to the DASH diet. I would love to hear what made you decide to try out the DASH diet. Is it to lower your blood pressure enough to finally rid yourself of blood pressure medication? Or perhaps to lose some weight due to health problems? Consider sharing your journey by leaving a short review on Amazon. It could have a positive impact on someone who is in the same situation.

CHAPTER THREE

Superstar Nutrients

Before we get into the recommended foods that make up the DASH diet, along with serving sizes and meal plans, we need to briefly look at the key nutrients that make DASH so effective in lowering blood pressure. This will help you understand why certain foods are recommended when we get to the food group section. DASH incorporates a wide variety of foods making it easy to follow since it doesn't require special foods or obscure ingredients you only find in specialized stores.

DASH is rich in whole grains, lean proteins, heart-healthy fats, low-fat dairy, beans, legumes, nuts, and seeds. Many of these foods are naturally high in fiber and essential minerals like potassium, calcium, and magnesium. These minerals are vital micronutrients and key positive players in managing blood pressure. When we break down each of them individually in this chapter, you will notice they have similar functions in the body. Potassium, calcium, and magnesium are all micronutrients known to help relax smooth muscles and reduce tension on your muscular blood vessels, which is why they are so beneficial to improving hypertension.[13]

Sodium

Let's start with "the bad" nutrient before we get to the good. As soon as anyone mentions blood pressure or hypertension, sodium comes into the conversation. Sodium has become the negative poster child for the high blood pressure problem we have in our country. On the one hand, sodium is an essential nutrient that the body needs. Unfortunately, on the other hand, it becomes a problem if there is too much sodium in the body. This can occur if you have kidney disease where the kidneys cannot get rid of excess sodium, or if you are salt-sensitive. But in most cases, our diets are to blame.

DASH recommends 2,300 mg of sodium a day, which may seem high for someone with hypertension. The average American consumes 3,440 mg of sodium per day,[14] so keeping it at 2,300 is a significant enough change to make a difference in your blood pressure. Breaking it down by gender, men average a daily intake of 4,240 mg while women average at 2,980 mg. However, research shows that anyone with hypertension who pairs the DASH diet with a low sodium intake of 1,500 mg, can lower blood pressure even more.[15] [16] So, it is worthwhile paying special attention to sodium in your meals.

But what is the difference between salt and sodium? Salt, or table salt, consists of 40% sodium and 60% chloride.[17] The recommended 2,300 mg of sodium equals about one teaspoon of salt (not tablespoon!). Next time you are in your kitchen, measure out a teaspoon of salt. You will notice that it doesn't look like a lot. The recommended amount of sodium for those with hypertension is 1,500 mg. To see what 1,500 mg of sodium looks like, measure out two-thirds of a teaspoon of table salt.

Salt is used excessively in packaged and processed foods. Bread, canned foods, pickles, soups, snacks, cured meats, and condiments contain quite a bit of sodium. These processed foods are responsible for up to 75% of daily sodium intake.[17] Thirty percent of sodium in your body is stored on the surface of your skeletal bones, and it is released into the bloodstream if your sodium levels drop. The rest of the sodium is found mostly in your plasma, as well as in the tissues of your nervous and muscular systems.

What if you decide to make a drastic statement by taking sodium out of your diet completely? Have you ever wondered to yourself, "Doing 0 mg of sodium should do the trick in lowering my blood pressure!" Don't do it, and here is why. Sodium is an electrolyte and is needed to manage your body's fluids, contract your muscles, aid in transmitting signals in your nervous system, and regulate your blood pressure, all of which would not be possible without Sodium.[18] The kidneys also help maintain the sodium balance by excreting excess sodium out of your body.

Why is sodium responsible for high blood pressure? How exactly does it work? If you ever cooked with zucchini or eggplant, you may have experienced salting these high-water-containing vegetables to reduce their water content. By adding salt, the sodium in the salt will extract the water out of the vegetable's plant cells and onto the surface. This process is how salt works in your bloodstream! Sodium is an ion that works outside of your cells and works to draw water and fluids into your bloodstream. If you have an excess amount of sodium in your system, it will surround your cells to carry more fluids into the bloodstream. This increase in blood volume results in higher blood pressure.[18]

Potassium

Another nutrient you may hear about is potassium, an electrolyte that helps perform similar functions in the body to sodium. Potassium regulates fluids and pH and helps send signals to the nervous system. It also helps with muscle contraction and maintains blood pressure by countering the effects of sodium.[19] This is the reason why a diet low in sodium and high in potassium is encouraged to lower blood pressure. Unlike sodium located outside of the body's cells, 95 to 98 percent of the potassium in your body is found inside the cells.

Various research has shown positive effects of potassium on blood pressure, even without lowering sodium.[20] [21] Increasing your intake of potassium by eating more unprocessed foods and incorporating plant-based foods into your meals can help reduce your systolic blood pressure by 4.4 mm Hg and lower your diastolic pressure by 2.5 mm Hg. Potassium helps lower your blood pressure by preventing the loss of calcium and magnesium, which are two micronutrients needed to relax your blood vessels. The current recommendation for potassium is 4,700 mg for adults,[22] a difficult number for many Americans to meet considering the average diet.

Potassium is in plant-based foods like fruits, vegetables, nuts, and legumes. Thus, meeting your potassium recommendation will be much easier under the DASH diet. In the following chapter, we will go over what foods contain potassium and how to get more of it in your daily diet!

Magnesium

Magnesium can potentially impact blood pressure in various ways. It can help relax muscles to release tension from your blood vessels. Cases of individuals with low magnesium resulted in tense muscles and increased blood pressure.[23] There have also been studies where individuals with high blood pressure have shown a more considerable amount of excreted magnesium, which means a decrease in retained magnesium. Magnesium is also needed to break down fats, which can be a factor in hypertension.[19]

So, perhaps we need more magnesium to lower blood pressure? Various studies have tried to test the relationship between magnesium and high blood pressure. Unfortunately, many of the results were inconclusive. Some trials were not well-controlled in their procedures, and with others the type and amount of magnesium supplements were inconsistent.[23] In analyzing these studies, some researchers found the possibility that magnesium might only be effective among people with magnesium deficiency, which could explain the inconsistent results.[24] Based on these findings and the potential positive effect magnesium could have on blood pressure, we recommend including magnesium-rich foods in your diet.

Calcium

Calcium is a major mineral and makes up 1.5 to 2 percent of our body weight. 99% of calcium is stored in our bones and teeth. The rest floats within the fluids inside and outside of our cells.[19] It is a common understanding that calcium plays a major role in bone health, but what might be surprising is its effects on heart health. Calcium is an electrolyte needed to contract muscles, make your heart beat and move blood, help your blood clot, and release hormones throughout your body.[18]

While these are core functions of calcium, why do so many people recommend calcium to reduce blood pressure? Instead of just joining the herd, we follow a research-based approach in our books, so here are our findings: Calcium's relation to blood pressure was first theorized in the 1970s, after observing a lower number of deaths from cardiovascular disease in communities with hard water (water with high calcium content). Since the 1990s, studies have tried to determine if calcium is beneficial for those with high blood pressure, with results being mainly inconclusive. Some studies showed positive effects, while others found it did not affect blood pressure whatsoever.[25 26 27]

Although calcium and hypertension data are inconclusive, there are a few theories on how calcium may be beneficial to blood pressure. It can help your muscles relax, which may reduce stress on your blood vessels. Also, calcium is affected by sodium and potassium. Having too much sodium in your body can cause you to lose calcium.[18] On the other hand, having more potassium in your body retains calcium and prevents loss.[19] This correlation might have an impact on blood pressure.

So, what does all this information mean to you and your diet? You should continue eating calcium-rich foods to maintain your health. But there is not enough data to support taking calcium supplements or trying to eat more calcium-rich foods than the recommended amount, just for the sake of lowering your blood pressure. For this reason, we take a mild approach to calcium.

Fiber

There is no way we can discuss nutrients without introducing fiber. Fiber is a big deal in the heart health world, yet it is not explicitly discussed as much with hypertension. It is a carbohydrate that is not digestible in the gastrointestinal tract. Instead, it helps move digested food out of your system. Some fiber will absorb water, and, as a bonus, some absorb dietary cholesterol and moves it out of your body. Fiber has shown that it can lower cholesterol levels and blood pressure, as well as reduce inflammation.[28] [29]

For this reason, we highly recommend including fiber in your meals. Fiber can be found in most plant-based foods. Therefore, increasing your intake of fruits, vegetables, whole grains, beans, legumes, nuts, and seeds with the DASH diet will naturally increase the amount of fiber you eat.

Nutrition can be complicated when we break it down to each nutrient to understand how they work, both individually and together, to help us overcome hypertension. Luckily, DASH makes nutrition easy by showing you exactly which foods to include for proper nutrition to lower your blood pressure, lose weight, and improve your overall health. This is exactly what we will look at, up next.

CHAPTER FOUR

Fabulous Food Groups of DASH

We have finally arrived at the DASH food groups. In this section, we will look at which foods to eat to get all the amazing nutrients we discussed in the previous chapter. We will thoroughly break down the DASH diet into its recommended food groups and learn about the different types of foods in each group. We will also look at the serving sizes for these foods. Then, in the next chapter, we will determine the ideal number of these servings for optimal weight loss, personalized to your physique and lifestyle.

The DASH diet does not exclude any major food groups. Instead, DASH follows an inclusive approach where it embraces all food groups, but it is concerned about the type of food included in each group. For example, it promotes whole grains over refined grains. With the DASH diet, you can have your carbohydrates and protein while pairing them with fruits and vegetables. Servings for dairy, fats, nuts, seeds, beans, and peas are achieved with balanced meals and snacks.

An important distinction to note in the upcoming sections is between servings and portions. A serving is a measurement of the food you are eating, while a portion is the total amount of food you eat at a sitting. For example, consider you have a cooked chicken breast that weighs about 3 ounces. According to DASH, one serving of chicken breast is 1 ounce. So, if you eat the whole chicken breast at a meal, then you have eaten three servings.

In the following sections, we will review what a serving size looks like for each food group. DASH serving sizes are slightly different from what you might be used to if you have followed any other diets in the past. So be sure to double-check serving sizes if you are in doubt. We also include a detailed quick reference table at the back of this book summarizing all food groups and serving sizes. Let's now take a look at the individual food groups to understand what nutrition they offer and what foods are available in each one. As you review each food group, note your favorite foods from each category, which will become part of your grocery list later!

Whole Grains

A grain derives from barley, oats, rice, wheat, oatmeal, and cereal grains. You are eating grains when you eat food products such as tortillas, pasta, bread, rice, popcorn, cereal, barley, oats, and quinoa. While carbohydrates with grains may be labeled as "unhealthy" in various fad diets, grains provide you with many nutrients. They are a good source of B vitamins, fiber, iron, antioxidants, and magnesium.[30] The B vitamins found in carbohydrates are essential in helping your body produce energy, which is a reason why carbs are a preferred source of energy compared to protein and fats.

In the DASH diet, grains are a heart-healthy food source, but you want to include mostly whole grains and reduce refined grains as much as possible. To understand why we pick whole grains, we will briefly discuss the makeup of a grain. A grain has three parts: an outer layer called the bran, an inner part called the endosperm, and a tiny spot inside called the germ. Each part holds different nutrients. The bran is the primary source of fiber, as well as minerals, B vitamins, and antioxidants. The endosperm makes up carbohydrates and protein. Lastly, the germ is responsible for growing new grains and is very nutritious with healthy fats, minerals, B vitamins, vitamin E, and antioxi-dants.[30]

Whole grains have all these layers intact. Thus, all the nutrients are intact as well. On the other hand, refined grains lose the nutritious bran and germ when it gets processed. The result is a grain made of just carbohydrates and protein. The fiber, vitamins, and minerals are gone. Whole grains will taste slightly different than refined grains and can be chewier in texture. The following are examples of whole-grain products: brown and wild rice, whole wheat or whole-grain corn tortillas, old-fashioned and steel-cut oats, whole wheat bread, pasta, English muffins, breakfast cereals, crackers, and bagels.

Food companies use refined grains to increase shelf life and soften their texture. Many companies attempt to add fiber, vitamins, and minerals by enriching or fortifying the refined grains, which you can see when looking at the ingredients listed on the nutrition label.[31] Refined grains can often be associated with added sugar and saturated fats, especially in products like muffins and pastries. Examples of refined grains are doughnuts, pancakes, flour tortillas, white rice, saltines, sourdough bread, plain bagels, corn flakes, and enriched pasta.

As you can see, whole grains are highly nutritious and is an integral part of a balanced diet. Moving forward with the DASH diet, make the majority of the grains you eat whole grains. Half a cup of cooked whole grains, such as rice, oats, corn, wheat, or quinoa, is equal to one serving. So too is half a cup of cooked pasta.

When looking at bread, any bread, bagel, English muffin, or roll the size of a slice of bread, is equal to one serving. Finally, one ounce of dry cereal or crackers is also one serving.[32] For packaged or processed grains like bread and pasta, look for a whole wheat or whole-grain variety. It should contain less than 140 mg of sodium per serving and have at least 3 grams of fiber. Double-check the ingredients in the nutrition label for whole-grain ingredients and avoid refined grains.

Whole grains cheat sheet

Serving Sizes	1/2 cup cooked whole grains or pasta.
	1 ounce dry cereal or crackers.
	1 slice of bread.
	1 small tortilla.
Recommended Foods	**Whole Grains**
	Amaranth, barley, brown rice, buckwheat, bulgur, corn kernels, couscous, farro, freekeh, kaniwa, kamut, millet, oats, orzo, psyllium, quinoa, rye, sorghum, spelt, teff, triticale, wheat, wild rice.
	Processed Whole Grains
	Bagels, bread, cereal, corn tortillas, crackers, English muffins, pasta, popcorn, rolls.

Vegetables

We know we need to eat our veggies, and there is a good reason for it. They are fantastic sources of vitamins, minerals, and fiber, which are all required nutrients to help your body be and stay healthy. The nutrients found in vegetables can prevent many diseases and health problems.

They are naturally low in calories and of course, cholesterol-free, which makes them great examples of nutrient-dense foods. We are always encouraged to "eat the rainbow" and ensure the vegetables on our plates have a variety of colors. While it is fun to say you ate the rainbow, there is a scientific explanation for this promotion. Specific plant colors contain specific nutrients. The nutrients you get from leafy greens are different from your red and yellow veggies. So, to get a decent combination of vitamins and minerals, you should eat a variety of different colored veggies.

Dark, green vegetables, such as spinach, kale, broccoli, collard greens, and romaine are good sources of vitamin K, potassium, folate, calcium, and magnesium. Red, yellow, and orange veggies like bell peppers, pumpkins, tomatoes, sweet potatoes, and squash are high in vitamins A, C, and folate.[18] With starchy vegetables, we don't need to look at their colors. Corn, peas, and potatoes fall in this category and are considered complex carbohydrates filled with potassium, zinc, and vitamin B6.[18] Beans, peas, and other legumes are also examples of vegetables, but some are categorized under the Nuts, Seeds, and Beans section.

In terms of the DASH diet, vegetables are the best way to help you meet your potassium recommendations. As we mentioned in the previous chapter, potassium is vital to help lower blood pressure. If you are looking into weight loss, adding more vegetables to your plate is a must. They are naturally lower in calories but contain enough fiber to still help you feel full. Thus, having more vegetables in your daily diet will help lower both your blood pressure and your weight! One serving size of vegetables equals one cup of any raw, leafy greens like spinach, romaine, kale, or collard greens. For cut vegetables, either raw or cooked, half a cup will count as a serving. The same goes for vegetable juice, half a cup equals one serving.[32] If vegetables are frozen or canned, opt for unsalted.

Vegetables cheat sheet

Serving Sizes	1 cup raw leafy greens. 1/2 cup cut, raw or cooked vegetables. 1/2 cup vegetable juice.
Recommended Foods	**Leafy Greens** Arugula, beet greens, bibb lettuce, broccoli rabe (rapini), butter lettuce, chicory, collard greens, dandelion greens, endive, iceberg lettuce, kale, mustard greens, Napa cabbage, red leaf lettuce, romaine lettuce, spinach, Swiss chard, turnip greens, watercress. **Squash and Gourds** Acorn, amber, ambercup, arikara, autumn cup, banana squash, bitter melon, buttercup, butternut, calabaza, carnival, chayote, crookneck, cucumber, cushaw, delicata, gem, gold nugget, hubbard, Jarrahdale pumpkin, kabocha, lakota, mooregold, patty pan, pumpkin, red kuri, spaghetti squash, sugar loaf, sweet dumpling, turban, yellow squash, yellow zucchini, zucchini. **Cruciferous Vegetables** Bok choy, broccoli, Brussels sprouts, cauliflower, green cabbage, red cabbage, radish, savoy cabbage, turnips.

Recommended Foods	**Legumes**
	Alfalfa, green beans, lentils, snow peas, sugar snap peas.
	Root Vegetables
	Arrowroot, beets, carrots, cassava. celery root, daikon, fennel, ginger, horseradish, jicama, kohlrabi, lotus root, parsnip, red onion, red potato, Russet potato, rutabaga, shallots, sweet onion, sweet potato, taro, white onion, yam root, yellow onion.
	Others
	Artichoke. asparagus, bell pepper, celery, corn on the cob, eggplant, heart of palm, leeks, mushroom, okra, radicchio, tomatillo, tomatoes.

Fruit

When we hear that we need to eat more fruit and veggies, we can always count on fruit being easy to increase, since fruit is nature's candy and are naturally tasty. When considering what source of fruit you want to add to your grocery list, consider whole fruits, which will contain all of their vitamins, minerals, and fiber. These are all nutrients essential in lowering the risks of diseases and for bettering our health. Whole fruits include the entire fresh fruit itself, cut up, dried, frozen, canned, and pureed.[18] Fruit juices made with 100% fruit (preferably with pulp) are also labeled as whole fruit.

Fruit cheat sheet

Serving Sizes	1/2 cup fresh, frozen, or canned fruit.
	1 medium-sized fruit.
	1/4 cup dried fruit.
	1/2 cup fruit juice.
Recommended Foods	**Berries** Blackberries, blueberries, boysenberries, cranberries, elderberries, gooseberries, loganberries, mulberries, raspberries, strawberries.
	Citrus Clementine, grapefruit, kumquat, lemon, lime, mandarin oranges, nectarine, orange, pomelo, tangerine.
	Tropical Avocado, banana, breadfruit, coconut meat, custard apple, dragon fruit, guava, durian, fig, jackfruit, kiwi, longan, lychee, mangoes, mangosteen, papaya, passion fruit, persimmon, pineapple, pomegranate seeds, rambutan, soursop, starfruit, sugar-apple, watermelon.
	Others Apples, apricots, Asian pear, blackcurrant, cantaloupe, cherimoya, cherries, dried fruit (no added sugar), grapes, honeydew, Medjool dates, olives, peaches, pears, plantain, plums, prickly pear, prunes, raisins (no added sugar).

Unfortunately, many juices and canned fruits have added sugar, which can be detrimental to your health and result in weight gain from the added calories. So, make sure you read the nutrition label to discover if those products contain any added sugars or syrup.

Fruit, in general, contain potassium, vitamin C, folate, fiber, and phytonutrients.[33] These nutrients are excellent for heart health, improving blood pressure, maintaining a healthy gastrointestinal tract, reducing cholesterol, healing wounds, and keeping your gums healthy. Like vegetables, fruit is naturally low in calories if eaten whole, making them a great addition to aid in weight loss. Fruit juice on the other hand can be deceptive. Due to the lack of fiber, you won't feel nearly as full, which can lead to over-consumption and easy weight gain. One glass of juice can easily contain the calories of 4 fruits.

Keep it exciting, and add a variety of fruit to your day. In addition to the typical apples, bananas, and oranges, find joy in adding berries, pomegranate seeds, Medjool dates, mangoes, pears, and papaya. One serving size of fruit equals half a cup of cut fruit, which can be fresh, frozen or canned, or one medium-sized fruit. The serving sizes for dried fruit and juices are smaller since they are much more concentrated than regular fruit, at one-quarter cup for dried fruit and half a cup for 100% fruit juices.[32] If you are on a statin medication, check with your doctor first before consuming grapefruit or grapefruit juice.

Dairy

While dairy is known for improving bone health thanks to its calcium content, it also provides riboflavin, potassium, vitamin B12, protein, magnesium, and phosphorus.[18] Vitamins A and D can also be found in yogurts and milk because dairy companies fortify them with those vitamins. Both the calcium and potassium content in dairy are beneficial to your blood pressure health.[34]

For the DASH diet, opt for low-fat or fat-free dairy products. Low-fat and fat-free products reduce the amount of fat content in dairy, which means they contain less saturated fats and calories. Dairy naturally contains sugar from lactose, but you can also find added sugars in dairies like flavored milk and yogurt. Checking the nutrition label for added sugars in the ingredients list will help you make a more informed decision when you are grocery shopping.

While calcium and potassium in dairy products are suitable for your health, keep in mind that cheese is a bit different from other dairies. Cheese is higher in calories due to its high content of cholesterol and fat, and tends to be high in sodium as well.[18] Always check the nutrition label to see how much sodium content is in a slice or ounce of cheese before buying it. Going for low-fat cheeses will help decrease the amount of fat, cholesterol, and calories.

The desire for sustainable and environmentally-friendly food sources has resulted in a rise in the popularity of plant-based milk such as soy, almond, coconut, oat, and macadamia milk.[35] Plant-based milk is a good alternative for those who are lactose-intolerant, vegetarian, vegan, or anyone who personally prefers milk substitutes over cow's milk. The nutrition varies amongst the types of plant-based milk, though in general, they tend to be more expensive and lower in protein than regular milk.[35]

Cow's milk also contains all the essential amino acids your body needs. Naturally, some milk alternatives can be a better source of heart-healthy fats and have been enriched and fortified with vitamins and minerals. Do check the nutrition labels as they may contain slightly more sodium and can contain added sugar. Look out for unsweetened versions of your favorite plant-based milk in the store. For reference, one serving of dairy is equal to one cup of either milk or yogurt, and 1.5 ounces of cheese.[32]

Dairy cheat sheet

Serving Sizes	1 cup milk. 1 cup yogurt. 1 1/2 ounces cheese.
Recommended Foods	**Dairy** Low-fat and fat-free plain milk, yogurt (no added sugar), and cheese. **Plant-Based** Calcium-fortified plant-based milk and yogurt (no added sugar). Plant-based made from almond, cashew, hemp, macadamia, oat, pea, or soy.

Meat, Poultry, and Fish

Meat, poultry, and fish are rich in amino acids but can be high in cholesterol and saturated fats, depending on the source. Animal-based protein and eggs provide all the amino acids you need for muscle building and are a good source of B12, which promotes nerve health. Protein is necessary for the health of our cells, hormones, and enzymes, and can also be converted into energy in dire situations.[36 37]

Vegetarian, vegan, and plant-based alternative protein sources include beans, lentils, peas, nuts, and seeds, as well as eggs in the case of vegetarians. Plant-based proteins offer only some of the amino acids our bodies need. Therefore, it is essential to eat multiple different food sources to get all the protein you need. Remember to swap out your animal-based protein servings from this food group for plant-based alternatives listed in the other food groups, if you follow a vegetarian, vegan, or plant-based lifestyle.

For those who prefer meat, poultry, and fish, opt for leaner sources that will be lower in saturated fats and calories. One strategy to find lean meats is to select meats with the USDA Select grade. USDA Select meats are low in marbling and fat.[38] You can also buy meats and trim the visible fat and remove excess skin. For fish, try to add a variety of fish to your diet including heart-healthy, fatty fish such as salmon, sardines, trout, and mackerel.

Proteins to exclude or to eat less often are those high in calories, saturated fats, cholesterol, and sodium. These include bacon, hot dogs, deli meats, sausage, ham, salami, chorizo, and corned beef.[18] Try swapping out these for some of the leaner options mentioned earlier. One serving size of cooked meat, poultry, or fish equals 1 ounce. While one egg or two egg whites are also one serving.[32]

Meat, poultry, and fish cheat sheet

Serving Sizes	1 ounce cooked meat, poultry, or fish. 1 egg or 2 egg whites.
Recommended Foods	**Meats** Canadian bacon, beef loin, beef round, ground beef (at least 90% lean), lamb leg, lamb loin, lamb rib, lamb shoulder, pork loin, pork round, veal rib, veal shoulder, venison, wild game. **Poultry** Chicken breast (skinless), egg, ground chicken, ground turkey, turkey. **Fish** Albacore tuna, flounder, herring, trout, mackerel, salmon, sardines, tilapia.

Fats and Oils

The low-fat diet craze has finally sizzled. We now understand that fats aid in absorbing essential vitamins, give us energy, keep us full, and are crucial for brain development and other body functions.[18] While we don't have to be scared of dietary fat anymore, we do need to educate ourselves on the type of fat we should eat. Particular fats can be heart-healthy, or they can contribute to heart disease. Let's discover the differences between the two.

Good fats are monounsaturated fats (MUFAs) and polyunsaturated fats (PUFAs). MUFAs and PUFAs are associated with better heart health since they don't raise our LDL cholesterol ("bad" cholesterol).[18] They are typically in liquid form at room temperature and include olive, canola, corn, walnut, sesame, and avocado oils. In terms of food, heart-healthy fats are in avocados, nuts, nut butter, and olives. Fish like salmon and tuna are also good sources of fats, specifically omega-3 and omega-6 fatty acids.

Fats and oils cheat sheet

Serving Sizes	1 teaspoon oil or other liquid fats. 1 teaspoon margarine or butter. 2 tablespoons low-fat salad dressing. (or 1 tablespoon regular dressing)
Recommended Foods	**Heart-Healthy Fats** Margarine (soft or liquid), salad dressings, sunflower seed butter, vegetable oil spread. **Oils** Avocado, canola, olive, peanut, safflower, soybean, walnut.

Fats to watch out for are saturated fats, trans fats, and partially hydrogenated oils. These fats can increase your LDL cholesterol which contributes to heart disease,[39][40] and should thus be eaten at a minimum. They tend to be solid at room temperature and can be found in butter, coconut and palm oils, lard, animal fat, and cheese. Nutrition labels should list the types of fats found in their products. This will make it easy to spot products with good fats and bad fats. One teaspoon of oil or other liquid fats equals one serving, the same goes for one teaspoon of margarine or butter. 2 tablespoons of low-fat salad dressing, or 1 tablespoon regular dressing, also equals one serving.[32]

Nuts, Seeds, Beans, and Peas

Legumes are highly nutritious and a great source of protein, fiber, potassium, iron, folate, magnesium, and phosphorus.[18] Most of these nutrients play a vital role in the DASH diet, which we discussed in the previous chapter. So, if you haven't tried many beans before, now might be the best time. You may be surprised which ones you end up liking! Legumes include lentils, chickpeas, black beans, kidney beans, split peas, peas, and pinto beans. Beans also have a chewy, meaty texture that makes a great meat alternative if you are interested in creating a few plant-based meals.

Nuts and seeds are packed with nutrients. They are a good source of vitamins and minerals, protein, and fiber, as well as antioxidants. Nuts are also heart-healthy as they contain MUFAs and PUFAs, while many seeds are high in omega-3 fatty acids.[18] Nuts and seeds are tasty and crunchy, making them fantastic additions to salads, yogurt, oatmeal, granola, or to be eaten as a snack. Explore different nuts and seeds such as almonds, walnuts, pistachios, macadamias, pecans, chia and flax seeds, as well as pumpkin, hemp, sesame, and sunflower seeds.

Nuts, seeds, beans, and peas cheat sheet

Serving Sizes	1/2 cup cooked legumes. 2 tablespoons nut butter. 1/3 cup or 1 1/2 ounces nuts. 2 tablespoons or 1/2 ounce seeds. 1/2 cup tofu.
Recommended Foods	**Nuts** Almond, almond butter, Brazil nut, cashew, cashew butter, chestnut, hazelnut, macadamia, Marcona almond, peanut, peanut butter, pecan, pili nut, pine nut, pistachio, tiger nut, walnut. **Seeds** Chia, flax, hemp, jackfruit seed, papaya seed, poppy, pumpkin seed, sesame, squash seed, watermelon seed, sunflower. **Peas** English peas, green peas, split peas. **Beans** Adzuki, black, black-eyed, cannellini, chickpea (garbanzo), cranberry, edamame, fava, Great Northern, kidney, lima, mung, pinto, navy, white, yellow, soybeans, and tofu.

Be wary of overindulging is nuts though. Due to their fat content, they are calorically dense foods and can rack up calories quickly without you noticing.

For reference, half a cup of cooked beans or peas equals a single serving. While 2 tablespoons of nut butter, such as peanut butter or almond butter, are also a serving. The same goes for seeds where 2 tablespoons equal a serving. Looking at nuts, a single serving is equal to one-third of a cup. For packaged products, opt for unsalted and unseasoned beans, nuts, nut butter, and seeds.[32]

Sweets and Treats

Going on the DASH diet doesn't mean you have to give up your favorite desserts, it just means you should enjoy them in moderation and smaller portions. The sweets and treats category includes general desserts, sodas, candy, sugary coffee drinks, ice cream, sports and energy drinks, and juices that are not 100% fruit. One serving size is about half a cup of ice cream, one ounce of cake, eight ounces of soda, two squares of milk chocolate, or 20 plain M&Ms.

With weight loss in mind, it's best to limit sweets and treats as much as possible, that's why we don't have any specific recommendations in this category. It would be ideal to eliminate sugary treats, but having an allowance for a few per week allows you to have a mental break from the diet, without going off completely. So, eat or drink your sweets slowly, and savor the flavor.

Building a DASH-friendly Plate

The breakdown of the DASH diet looked at the different food groups with their recommended serving sizes. It focused on the type of foods from each group to best promote heart health and improve hypertension. Take a moment to reflect on your nutrition and see what areas you excel at and which areas you can improve on. Remember that little changes can make a big difference.

Keeping track of serving sizes for all the different food groups every day can be a bit intimidating at first, but the more you practice building a DASH-friendly plate, the easier it will be. Nutrition is also not an exact science, so being a little off with serving sizes here and there is not the end of the world. Every meal will look a little different. The most important part of any diet change is consistency. Being aware of what you eat and making a conscious effort to add more fruits, vegetables, whole grains, and lean protein to your diet is the first step to success.

In the next chapter, we will find out exactly how many servings of each food group you should include in your meals to start shedding those pounds! To help you on your DASH journey, we include a wonderful 21-day customizable meal plan in Chapter 6, that allows you to mix and match meals depending on your appetite and the contents of your fridge. We also include 30 flavorful recipes, that cover everything from Caribbean jerk shrimp to chocolate peanut butter smoothies in Chapter 14.

CHAPTER FIVE

Implementing DASH

In this chapter, we'll show you how the standard DASH diet can be tailored to promote healthy weight loss, while remaining true to everything that makes DASH so great. We will also address other aspects that should be considered when implementing the DASH diet, such as salt- and food-substitutes, cooking techniques, and how to overcome the perils of dining out while on a diet. Let's start with the most burning question first: "How exactly can I lose weight with DASH?"

DASH for Weight Loss

To lose weight with DASH is a simple two-step process. First, we will determine how many calories you need for optimal healthy weight loss. Don't worry, we will not be counting calories or tracking macros! Then, we will use this calorie number to choose a DASH plan that best suits you.

Step 1 – Choosing Your Daily Calories

The science behind weight loss is pretty straightforward but can be a mine-field of math and formulas. In simple terms, to lose weight your caloric intake (what you eat) needs to be less than what your body requires in a day. By having this calorie deficit, your body will seek other forms of energy and start to tap into your fat stores.

This usually requires you to know your Basal Metabolic Rate (BMR) and Total Daily Energy Expenditure (TDEE). BMR is the amount of energy your body needs to function at rest, or in other words if you did absolutely nothing. Think of someone in a coma. Their body will still require nutrients for breathing, digestion, blood circulation, brain function, etc.

TDEE is the number of calories you burn during the day as a result of your daily physical activities, such as your job and how often you work out. This is done by adjusting BMR by an activity factor. This final number is then reduced by a static number or percentage to obtain your ideal caloric intake for weight loss.

If all of this sounds like a headache, don't worry, we have already done all these calculations for you and compiled the results in a neat, easy-to-follow table on the following pages. Simply choose the table for women or men, then your age range, current weight, and current activity level. The activity levels are defined as follows:

❀ **Sedentary**   Little to no exercise and no physically demanding job.

❀ **Lightly Active**   Working out or playing sports 1–3 days per week.

❀ **Moderately Active**   Working out or playing sports 3–5 days per week.

❀ **Very Active**   Working out or playing sports 6–7 days per week.

Daily calorie requirements for weight loss (women)

Age	Weight (lbs.)	Sedentary	Lightly Active	Moderately Active	Very Active
19 - 29	up to 139	1200	1300	1500	1600
	140 - 159	1200 – 1300	1300 – 1400	1500 – 1600	1600 – 1700
	160 - 199	1300 – 1400	1400 – 1600	1600 – 1800	1700 – 1900
	200 - 239	1400 – 1600	1600 – 1700	1800 – 2000	1900 – 2100
	240+	1600	1700	2000	2100
30 - 39	up to 139	1100	1200	1400	1500
	140 - 159	1100 – 1200	1200 – 1300	1400 – 1500	1500 – 1600
	160 - 199	1200 – 1400	1300 – 1500	1500 – 1700	1600 – 1800
	200 - 239	1400 – 1500	1500 – 1700	1700 – 1900	1800 – 2000
	240+	1500	1700	1900	2000

Daily calorie requirements for weight loss (women)

Age	Weight (lbs.)	Sedentary	Lightly Active	Moderately Active	Very Active
40 – 49	up to 139	1100	1200	1400	1500
	140 – 159	1100 – 1200	1200 – 1300	1400 – 1500	1500 – 1600
	160 – 199	1200 – 1300	1300 – 1500	1500 – 1600	1600 – 1800
	200 – 239	1300 – 1500	1500 – 1600	1600 – 1800	1800 – 2000
	240+	1500	1600	1800	2000
50+	up to 139	1100	1200	1300	1400
	140 – 159	1100 – 1200	1200 – 1300	1300 – 1400	1400 – 1500
	160 – 199	1200 – 1300	1300 – 1400	1400 – 1600	1500 – 1700
	200 – 239	1300 – 1500	1400 – 1600	1600 – 1800	1700 – 1900
	240+	1500	1600	1800	1900

Daily calorie requirements for weight loss (men)

Age	Weight (lbs.)	Sedentary	Lightly Active	Moderately Active	Very Active
19 – 29	up to 170	1500	1700	1900	2000
	170 – 200	1500 – 1700	1700 – 1800	1900 – 2000	2000 – 2200
	200 – 230	1700 – 1800	1800 – 1900	2000 – 2200	2200 – 2300
	230 – 260	1800 – 1900	1900 – 2100	2200 – 2300	2300 – 2500
	260+	1900	2100	2300	2500
30 – 39	up to 170	1500	1600	1800	2000
	170 – 200	1500 – 1600	1600 – 1800	1800 – 2000	2000 – 2100
	200 – 230	1600 – 1700	1800 – 1900	2000 – 2100	2100 – 2300
	230 – 260	1700 – 1900	1900 – 2000	2100 – 2300	2300 – 2400
	260+	1900	2000	2300	2400

Daily calorie requirements for weight loss (men)

Age	Weight (lbs.)	Sedentary	Lightly Active	Moderately Active	Very Active
40 – 49	up to 170	1500	1600	1800	1900
	170 – 200	1500 – 1600	1600 – 1700	1800 – 1900	1900 – 2100
	200 – 230	1600 – 1700	1700 – 1800	1900 – 2100	2100 – 2200
	230 – 260	1700 – 1800	1800 – 2000	2100 – 2200	2200 – 2400
	260+	1800	2000	2200	2400
50+	up to 170	1400	1600	1800	1900
	170 – 200	1400 – 1500	1600 – 1700	1800 – 1900	1900 – 2000
	200 – 230	1500 – 1700	1700 – 1800	1900 – 2000	2000 – 2200
	230 – 260	1700 – 1800	1800 – 1900	2000 – 2200	2200 – 2400
	260+	1800	1900	2200	2400

Let's look at an example. If Jane is a 35-year-old woman, that weighs 190 pounds, and is not physically active, her recommended calories to lose weight will be 1,200 to 1,400 per day. This means that if she ate no more than 1,200 to 1,400 calories every day, she will lose weight. Go ahead and look up your own recommended calorie number right now. We'll use this number in step two.

For those who love science and math, we calculated the caloric ranges using the Mifflin-St Jeor Equation as this was found to be the most accurate and reliable.[41] We used activity multipliers from Michael Matthews rather than the more widely-used Harris-Benedict multipliers. The Harris-Benedict activity factors tend to overestimate caloric requirements.[42][43] And lastly, we applied a 20% deficit, which was found to be ideal for optimal fat loss without the downsides of losing lean muscle and negatively impacting metabolism.[44]

Step 2 – Choosing a DASH Plan

Now that you have your ideal number of daily calories to lose weight, we'll choose a matching DASH diet plan. The National Institutes of Health (NIH) prescribes guidelines for daily servings of the various DASH food groups.[32] These guidelines tell us exactly how many servings of each food group we need per day, based on predefined calorie requirements. The guidelines are shown below and are for nine calorie groupings ranging from 1,200 calories to 2,800 calories.

Based on your ideal daily calories determined in step one, choose the closest matching calorie group from the table. If your recommended calories span across two groups, choose the group based on where you fall on the weight range in step one. For instance, in our earlier example, Jane's recommended calorie number was 1,200 to 1,400 per day. But we have DASH plans for both those numbers. If you recall, Jane weighs 190 pounds, placing her on the upper end of the 160 - 199 pound range (from the table in step 1).

She would then choose the higher 1,400 calorie group. In this group, Jane would aim for 5 to 6 servings of whole grains per day, 3 to 4 servings of vegetables per day, 4 servings of fruit per day, and so on. Go ahead and choose your DASH plan right now. Your plan will prescribe exactly how many servings of each food group you need per day. The recommended servings are presented as daily servings unless stated otherwise.

You now know exactly how many servings of each food group you need per day for sustained weight loss on the DASH diet. You also know the recommended size of those servings and which foods are included in each food group, from the previous chapter. The sodium recommendation above is 2,300 mg per day for all categories. But as we discussed in Chapter 3, research has found that lowering to 1,500 mg per day can result in a more significant decrease in blood pressure.[15][16] We do recommend aiming for 1,500 mg if you have severely high blood pressure.

Notice also the weekly allotment of sweets and treats. Excluding sweets and treats completely can lead to feelings of guilt if you "break" your meal plan, which can quickly spiral out of control when a cheat meal becomes a cheat day. A better approach is allowing for a few sweets and treats throughout the week, which satisfies cravings while still keeping you on your DASH goals of lowering blood pressure and losing weight. While the DASH diet allows sweets and treats, our goal is still healthy weight loss. So, approach this food group cautiously.

Now that you know exactly how many servings of each DASH food group you need per day for healthy sustained weight loss, we'll look at a few other aspects that you should consider when implementing DASH.

DASH plans (daily servings per food group)

Daily calories	1,200	1,400	1,600	1,800	2,000	2,200	2,400	2,600	2,800
Whole grains	4 – 5	5 – 6	6	6	6 – 8	8 – 9	9 – 10	10 – 11	11 – 12
Vegetables	3 – 4	3 – 4	3 – 4	4 – 5	4 – 5	4 – 5	5 – 6	5 – 6	5 – 6
Fruit	3 – 4	4	4	4 – 5	4 – 5	5	5 – 6	5 – 6	5 – 6
Dairy	2 – 3	2 – 3	2 – 3	2 – 3	2 – 3	3	3	3	3
Meat, poultry and fish	3 or less	4 or less	4 or less	6 or less	6 or less	6 or less	6 or less	6 or less	6 – 9
Fats and oils	1	1	2	2 – 3	2 – 3	2 – 3	3	3	3 – 4
Nuts, seeds, beans & peas	3 per week	3 per week	3-4 pr week	4 per week	4-5 pr week	5-6 pr week	5-6 pr week	7 per week	7 per week
Sweets and treats	3 or less per week								
Sodium	2,300 mg								

DASH Substitutes

Since processed foods contain a large amount of sodium, one of the best ways to reduce your sodium intake is to cook at home using fresh ingredients. This allows you to select lean proteins and whole grains, and to purchase your favorite fruits and vegetables. By preparing your meals, you have total control over the amount of salt used in your food. Not only that, but you also have control over the sugars, fats, and calories you eat, kicking your weight loss into high gear!

A big part of the DASH diet is reducing your sodium intake. Cutting out sodium might seem difficult to do in your daily life, but it doesn't need to be. Start slowly by first decreasing your portions of high sodium snacks and foods. Having a strong preference for salty foods is an acquired taste and can be adjusted over time. As you start eating less salty snacks and lessen salt in your cooking, your taste buds will eventually prefer foods lower in sodium.

Salt Substitutes

There are many different types of salt on the market, with some being seen as healthier than others. Whether you are reaching for pink Himalayan salt, iodized salt, or sea salt, when it comes to sodium - salt is salt. No matter the type, all salt should be measured towards your daily intake of sodium.

A few shakes of the salt shaker can add 300 to 600 mg of sodium to a meal.[18] Before reaching for the table salt to season your food, taste it first. If it already has flavor, skip the salt. Otherwise, try flavoring your food with herbs, a squeeze of citrus, black pepper, and other spices. There are a lot of flavor combinations you can discover that require little or no salt! Another strategy you can try is to cook with no salt and add just a bit of salt over the food before serving.

For salt substitutes, some people recommend substitutes that contain potassium chloride (KCl), which looks like salt and can taste like it too. We highly recommend not using these types of substitutes, unless approved by your doctor. Potassium chloride may cause adverse effects for people on certain medications for hypertension and other heart diseases.[45] The excessive potassium from these salt substitutes can also be harmful to anyone with chronic kidney disease.[46]

Since salt substitutes can be hazardous, depending on your situation, we recommend going for herb blends with no added salt. Be sure to read the nutrition labels of bottled herbs and spices to see if it contains any sodium. If you don't find any blends you like in-store, you can create your own. Some examples of our favorite herb blends are Italian, curry, Mexican, and Chinese five-spice. Herb blends may not taste like salt, but they come packed with flavor!

Salt cheat sheet

Serving Sizes	1 teaspoon salt = 2,325 mg sodium
Flavor Alternatives	Basil, balsamic vinegar, black pepper, cayenne, chili, cilantro, chives, cinnamon, cumin, garlic, garlic powder, lemon juice, lemon zest, lime juice, lime zest, onion, orange zest, paprika, parsley, red pepper flakes, rosemary, thyme, vinegar

Food Substitutes

Swapping out other ingredients in a recipe is a good strategy for reducing calories, saturated fats, and added sugar. This will not only make a big difference in your blood pressure but also your weight loss efforts. The idea is to swap less-healthy ingredients in your existing recipes and meals with some-thing more nutritious from the DASH food groups, containing fiber, vitamins, minerals, extra protein, or heart-healthy fats. This way any home-cooked meal can be a DASH meal!

For instance, swap bacon for Canadian bacon, which is flavorful yet contains significantly less sodium. For ground beef, select 90 percent or higher lean op-tions, or swap for ground turkey or beans. Use Greek yogurt over buttermilk or sour cream. Instead of croutons on a salad, substitute with nuts, seeds, bean sprouts, or crunchy cucumbers and carrots. Suppose a fried rice recipe calls for white rice, use brown rice instead. Or if a smoothie recipe adds sugar, rather opt for a Medjool date or a ripe banana.

We always recommend using fresh produce. But if you are in a situation where you feel you want to incorporate canned or frozen produce, go for items with no added salt. We also strongly advise reducing ingredients such as ham, bologna, pickles, olives, and bacon.

These items are surprisingly high in sodium. To give you an idea of how much sodium these ingredients have, check out the numbers: Two slices of ba-con contain about 360 mg of sodium, five olives from a bottle have 210 mg, a slice of bologna has 850 mg, and one slice of ham contains 960 mg![47] Once you advance your cooking skills, you can also minimize the use of pre-packaged sauces and salad dressings and make them from scratch instead.

Healthy Cooking Techniques

When deciding how to cook your food, we recommend opting for techniques that require very little oil. Instead of deep-fried foods, go for baked or grilled options. Fat has a higher calorie content per gram than protein or carbohy-drates (9 calories per gram vs 4), so reducing fat can significantly lower your calorie intake without making too much of a difference in how much you eat.

We do however still need fat in our diet to absorb different types of vitamins in our bodies, so choose heart-healthy oils like grape seed and avocado oils to cook with at home. These are much healthier than using lard or butter, which contain saturated fats.

Baking and grilling are among the healthiest techniques for preparing food, but they aren't your only options. Fish can be steamed or poached. Veggies can be steamed, sautéed, boiled, or pan-fried with a small amount of plant-based oil. Poultry and meat can be roasted, stewed, or pan-fried similar to veggies. Roasting and stir-fries are also excellent ways to "clean out" your fridge before you need to restock. When working with poultry and meat, remember to trim any visible fat and remove the skin. If you see visible oil or grease after cooking, dab it with a paper towel to remove any excess.

With technology advancing all around us, the kitchen is no exception. Many kitchen gadgets have made cooking simple and healthier. Steamers, air fryers, pressure cookers, and indoor grills can all help you prepare your favorite proteins, fruits, and vegetables easily while reducing the need for oil. If you are inexperienced in the kitchen, don't worry! Later in this book, we will go over basic cooking techniques to help you on your journey, along with 30 delicious recipes that are easy to follow.

Tips for Eating Out

While the DASH diet is best if you eat out less, many of us enjoy spending time with family and friends when dining out. So, here we will share some tips you can follow to select the best menu items that fit your DASH goals when you do go out to restaurants.

If you go out to eat once in a blue moon for specific occasions, enjoy the meal and eat whatever you desire. Follow mindful eating techniques, and come back to your DASH principles the next day. If you eat out quite often, whether it is for work, social occasions, or because it is a frequent alternative to preparing meals at home, check out these tips. It's important to note that foods from restaurants, fast-casual chains, and fast-food spots tend to be high in sodium, fat, and sugar. Portion sizes are also much more substantial than recommended.

Interpreting the Menu

Many major restaurants and fast-food chains post nutritional info for their meals online. An online search for the restaurant name, followed by the word "nutrition" should work. This way, you can make DASH-friendly selections before you ever step foot in the restaurant. The nutrition information will generally list calories, saturated fats, sodium, fiber, and sugar. Some may contain information on vitamins and minerals. Either way, look out for foods low in saturated fats, sodium, and sugar, and high in fiber and potassium.

Particular cooking techniques like curing meat and brining use a lot of salt, and some sauces also contain a sizable amount of sodium. Luckily, you can usually spot these on the menu by recognizing a few different terms. Menu items with teriyaki, cocktail, soy, and Creole sauces are high in sodium.[18] Anything pickled, marinated, smoked, cured, au jus, or barbecued are also high-sodium indicators.[18] Skipping these items is recommended to keep your sodium intake below the recommended amount.

Items high in fat and calories are typically breaded, deep-fried, or served with creamy sauces. Sometimes you will find these keywords in the menu name itself or the item's description. The following are keywords for fried foods: crispy, batter-fried, deep-fried, french-fried, and lightly fried.[18] High-calorie sauces are in menu items containing aioli, smothered, hollandaise, buttered, creamy, gravy, beurre blanc, cream sauce, scalloped, bearnaise, and cheese sauce.[18] If you would like to enjoy these sometimes, ask for the sauce on the side so you can lightly dip your food in it. It will give you more control over how much you consume.

So, what should you look for on the menu that can align with your DASH goals? Similar to the healthy cooking techniques we mentioned earlier, restaurants that practice similar styles will reflect it in the food's description. Opt for protein and veggies with the following keywords: stir-fried, poached, grilled, broiled, braised, baked, steamed, roasted, or sauteed.[18] These will be lean options you can find at a restaurant in terms of fat and calories, but they will not guarantee a low sodium content. You can check the menu's online nutritional information or ask the waiter if the cooks can make the meals without salt.

Other Considerations

Practice mindful eating and portion control. Eat slowly, enjoy the company around you, savor the flavor, and eat until you are comfortably full. Once you are satisfied, pack up the rest of the food in a to-go container, which becomes a second meal for later. You can also split a meal with someone else if the restaurant allows it.

To lower calories, order your sauces, condiments, and salad dressings on the side, and choose lean cuts of protein. Balance your meal when selecting side dishes for your entrees, such as steamed vegetables or whole grains. For dessert, angel food cake with fresh strawberries, sorbet, or assorted fruits are good options. If you find yourself at a buffet, use your plate as a visual guide to building a healthy dish. Fill up half of your plate with salad and vegetables, a quarter plate of protein, and the remainder with whole grains.

Drinks are often the reason a meal is so high in calories and sugar. Skip on the wine, cocktails, lemonade, shakes, and sodas. Water and unsweetened carbonated water are ideal for staying hydrated and are also favorable for your blood pressure. If you want some flavor, ask the waiter for a wedge of lemon. Black coffee and unsweetened tea are also good options.

DASH for Vegetarians and Vegans

As mentioned at the beginning of the guide, the DASH diet is practical and flexible for vegetarians and vegans. Most of the DASH guidelines will be applied the same, such as eating more fruits, vegetables, whole grains, nuts, seeds, legumes, and heart-healthy fats. Let's look at how your plate will look on the DASH diet.

For both vegetarians and vegans, you will swap out your animal-based protein servings for plant-based alternatives. Variety is key here! Each plant-based source provides different amino acids, so it is recommended to eat a range of plant-based proteins to ensure you get all the essential amino acids. Peas, lentils, beans, and other legumes, as well as soybeans, edamame, tempeh, textured vegetable protein, soy patties, soy cheese, and tofu, are good sources of protein.[48] Depending on which protein source you want to use, try them in stir-fries, pasta, tacos, pizza, chili, and formed into patties for a burger. Incorporating nuts and nut butter can easily add more protein to your diet.

For vegans, cutting out dairy and eggs should be no problem if you are incorporating the abovementioned plant-based protein sources. For calcium, you can opt for calcium-fortified products found in juice, plant-based milk, and cereal.[49] Being vegetarian or vegan can put you at risk for some nutrition deficiencies. Working with a Registered Dietitian is recommended to ensure you are optimizing your nutrition on a plant-based diet.

CHAPTER SIX

Custom Meal Plan

To help you get started with the DASH diet, this section provides DASH-friendly meal and snack suggestions. The meals are a combination of lean protein, whole grains, fruits, and vegetables. Standard meal plans force you to eat a specific meal at a specific time, but what if you don't have a required ingredient in your fridge or pantry, or you're simply not in the mood for chicken with a side salad for the third night in a row?

For this reason, we created a 21-day customizable meal plan. Pick and choose from the delicious suggestions below to build a personalized menu for yourself. You can get creative and combine meals from each group based on your taste and available ingredients. You have complete freedom! Just because a meal is listed as lunch doesn't mean you can't make it for dinner. All meals are 100% DASH approved and are varied enough so your taste buds won't get bored!

When preparing these meals, remember to follow the DASH guidelines for ingredients, serving sizes, salt substitutes, and cooking methods as set out in Chapters 4 and 5. Most important, remember to stick to the recommended number of servings we determined in Chapter 5 to ensure healthy sustained weight loss. Meals marked with page numbers have complete easy-to-follow recipes in Chapter 14.

Breakfast

Two-Egg Omelette
Omelette cooked in olive oil and filled with sauteed Canadian bacon, spinach, bell peppers, and onions.

Morning Toast
Whole grain toast, spread with almond butter, topped with sliced strawberries.

Breakfast Sandwich
Whole grain English muffin with one-egg scramble, arugula, and radish.

Savory Oatmeal (p132)
Nourishing, fiber-rich oats accompanied by protein-rich egg whites, creamy avocado, and bright sauteed peppers.

Morning Parfait
Layers of plain, nonfat Greek yogurt, sugar-free granola, and fresh berries.

Breakfast Tacos
Corn tortillas filled with scrambled eggs, corn, black beans, salsa, cilantro, and sliced avocado.

Raspberry Breakfast Muffin
Raspberry muffin made with rolled oats and whole wheat flour.

<u>Berries & Greens Smoothie</u> (p140)
Coconut milk blended with blueberries, strawberries, and kale, with a hint of honey, boosted with plant-based protein from hemp seeds.

<u>English Breakfast</u>
Sunny-side-up egg over whole-grain toast, served with pinto beans and seared cherry tomatoes.

<u>Cinnamon Apple Oatmeal</u>
Steel-cut oatmeal topped with walnuts and baked cinnamon apples.

<u>Tropical Pina Colada Smoothie</u> (p138)
Coconut milk paired with frozen pineapple chunks, protein-packed Greek yogurt, topped with unsweetened coconut flakes.

<u>Avocado Toast</u>
Whole grain toast with sliced avocado, cherry tomatoes, sprouts, and a poached egg.

<u>Berry Waffle</u>
Whole grain waffle topped with fresh berries, a dollop of plain, nonfat yogurt, and finished with lemon zest.

<u>Southwest Sweet Potato Hash</u> (p134)
Sweet and crispy sweet potatoes, protein-packed ground chicken and eggs, spinach for a micronutrient boost, and warm and flavorful spices.

Shakshuka

Eggs cooked over a base of unsalted, canned plum tomatoes, served with whole-grain bread.

Tropical Yogurt Bowl

Plain, nonfat yogurt topped with kiwi, mango, pomegranate seeds, and sugar-free granola.

Overnight Cherry Chia Oats

Rolled oats and chia seeds soaked overnight in unsweetened, vanilla almond milk, topped with pitted cherries, sliced almonds, and a drizzle of honey.

Veggie Tofu Scramble (p136)

An egg-less scramble loaded with plant-based protein, bell peppers, yellow onion, spinach, and a hint of turmeric.

Lemon Blueberry Pancakes

Lemon blueberry pancakes made with whole wheat flour and topped with fresh blueberries, plain, nonfat yogurt, lemon zest, and a sugar-free raspberry chia seed jam.

Chocolate Peanut Butter Smoothie (p139)

Oat milk blended with cocoa powder, peanut butter, and bananas.

Asian-Style Rice and Eggs

Two egg scramble with shrimp and scallions, served over brown rice and sauteed bok choy, topped with toasted sesame seeds, chopped cilantro, and a drizzle of Sriracha.

Lunch

Black Bean & Sweet Potato Tacos
Mix of black beans, sweet potatoes, peppers, and onions,
seasoned with taco seasoning and served in corn tortillas, topped
with salsa, cilantro, and shredded lettuce.

Chicken Marinara Sandwich
Grilled chicken breast topped with sauteed eggplant and onions,
between two slices of whole-grain bread, served with marinara
dip.

Chipotle Chicken Salad (p157)
Chicken breast with a smokey spice rub, paired with a healthy
homemade ranch dressing loaded with lemon juice and fresh
dill.

Black Bean Burger
Grilled black bean patty, with mustard, lettuce, tomatoes,
onions, and fresh jalapenos, served between a whole-grain bun,
with a butter lettuce salad.

Caribbean Jerk Shrimp (p144)
Jumbo shrimp covered with a punchy spice rub, served with
creamy coconut rice and sweet steamed peas.

Salmon Patties
Two salmon patties, lightly pan-fried and served over a bed of
arugula, red onions, and tomatoes tossed in a lemon vinaigrette.

Shredded Barbecue Chicken Bowl (p148)

Shredded chicken breast with a warm and smoky barbecue sauce, crunchy baked carrots, and chewy farro.

Chickpea Burger

Chickpea patty lightly pan-fried and topped with butter lettuce, sliced tomato, red onions, and guacamole, served in a whole wheat bun with a side of baked potato wedges.

Ginger Chicken Lettuce Wraps

Lettuce cups with sauteed ground chicken, ginger, carrots, peppers, scallions, topped with a light hoisin sauce and seasoning.

Sirloin & Veggie Kebabs (p188)

Skewered and grilled sirloin, onion, zucchini, and summer squash, with a rich and creamy garlic and yogurt dip.

Black Bean Quesadillas

Reduced-fat Mexican cheese blend, melted over a whole wheat tortilla, filled with black beans and fajita veggies.

Deconstructed Sushi Bowl

Salmon and diced onions cooked with low-sodium soy sauce, served over brown rice, edamame, julienned cucumbers and carrots, and seaweed, topped with sesame seeds.

Spaghetti Squash and Meatballs

Baked Italian chicken meatballs over spaghetti squash and marinara sauce, topped with basil.

Chickpea Salad Lettuce Wraps (p176)
Chickpeas with crisp celery, crunchy carrots, and tender pine nuts, wrapped in fresh lettuce with a tangy sauce.

Lentil Taco Salad
Tender lentils sauteed with low-sodium taco seasoning served over lettuce, tomatoes, red onions, fresh jalapeno, black beans, corn, avocado, salsa, and low-sodium corn chips.

Buffalo Turkey Burgers (p152)
Juicy turkey patties on a whole wheat bun, with tomato slices, cool cucumber, and crisp romaine with sweet potato fries.

Middle Eastern Lunch Box
Whole-grain pita with hummus spread, a side of tabbouleh salad, and a Medjool date.

Vegan Lentil Ragu with Spaghetti Squash (p182)
Spaghetti squash carrying a lentil-based ragu full of bright tomatoes, tender carrots, crisp celery, and punchy garlic and onions.

Loaded Baked Potato
Baked russet potato loaded with plain, nonfat yogurt, sauteed mushrooms, tomatoes, green onions, and reduced-fat shredded cheddar cheese.

Easy Lunch Box
Boiled egg, whole-grain bread with nut butter, baby carrots, and grapes.

Power Greens Salad (p162)

Massaged kale leaves with feta cheese, sweet dried cranberries, quinoa, and crunchy sunflower seeds, topped with a sweet and tangy honey mustard dressing.

Vietnamese Spring Rolls with Peanut Sauce

Vermicelli, boiled shrimp, cucumbers, bean sprouts, lettuce, mint leaves, and cilantro, wrapped in rice paper and dipped in peanut sauce.

Chicken and Rice

Diced roasted chicken breast over brown rice and steamed broccoli, with a squeeze of lemon juice.

Tofu Fried Rice

Fried brown rice, peas, carrots, corn, spinach, and cubed tofu, lightly seasoned with low-sodium soy sauce and Sriracha.

Summer Berry Salad (p160)

Juicy strawberries and blueberries, with creamy goat cheese, crunchy almonds, and punchy red onion, covered by a sweet strawberry vinaigrette.

Dinner

Mango Avocado Salsa Salmon (p146)

Oven-baked savory salmon and cilantro lime rice, with sweet mango and avocado salsa.

Tofu Strips
Grilled tofu strips over quinoa, arugula, and grilled zucchini, with a drizzle of lemon vinaigrette.

Veggie Loaded Chili (p166)
Crumbled ground chicken, fiber-filled black beans, tender sweet potatoes, and bell peppers, with tomatoes, warm chili powder and cumin.

Chicken Fajita Casserole (p150)
Casserole featuring tender chicken, sweet onions and bell peppers, warm aromatic spices, and protein-packed quinoa.

Spaghetti with Lentil Meatballs
Whole wheat spaghetti and lentil meatballs, tossed in low-sodium pasta sauce, with bell peppers, zucchini, and onions.

Honey Mustard Pork Tenderloin (p190)
Pork tenderloin, carrots, and golden potatoes, smothered in a creamy, sweet and punchy homemade honey mustard sauce.

Veggie Pesto Pizza
Bell peppers, onions, spinach, mushrooms, broccoli, basil, and pesto over whole wheat naan.

Vegan Tofu Stir Fry Bowl (p173)
Tofu, brown rice, and lots of vegetables, all swimming in a robust and flavorful stir-fry sauce with hints of garlic, ginger, chili, and sesame oil.

<u>Sirloin with Chimichurri Sauce</u> (p186)
Seared sirloin with asparagus and red onion, covered in a
homemade chimichurri sauce with hints of jalapeno, garlic,
cilantro, and parsley.

<u>Hawaiian BBQ Skewers</u>
Skewers with chickpea meatballs, red bell peppers, and
pineapple slices, lightly brushed with low-sodium BBQ sauce
and served over brown rice.

<u>Honey & Garlic Tempeh</u> (p180)
Tempeh dripping in a sticky honey and garlic glaze, with
crispy baked vegetable fries sprinkled with a simple spice blend
that complements the flavorful tempeh.

<u>Shredded Chicken Tortilla Soup</u> (p164)
Chicken breast, fiber-loaded brown rice and vegetables, with
a smooth and flavorful tomato broth, topped with crunchy
tortilla chips.

<u>Split Pea Fritters</u>
Pan-fried split pea fritters (split peas, onions, garlic, carrot,
zucchini, ground flaxseed, and whole wheat bread crumbs),
served over bibb lettuce dressed in lemon vinaigrette and black
pepper.

<u>Greek Grain Bowl</u> (p170)
Couscous and pickled onions, loaded with chickpeas,
cucumbers, and fresh cherry tomatoes, finished off with a
homemade dill-infused tzatziki dressing.

Chili Lime Baked Tilapia (p142)
Tilapia filets baked with a chili-lime spice rub, served on a bed of bok choy and sweet onions.

Shrimp Pasta Primavera
Whole wheat penne pasta, carrots, broccoli, yellow squash, cherry tomatoes, red bell pepper, zucchini, and shrimp, sauteed in olive oil and garlic, with a squeeze of lemon juice.

Herbed Chicken with Spicy Peanut Sauce (p154)
Herbed chicken breast with smooth and creamy peanut sauce, whole grains, crisp cucumbers, and roasted broccoli.

Baked Eggplant Parmesan
Baked eggplant parmesan made with reduced-fat parmesan and low-sodium tomato sauce, served over whole-grain spaghetti and steamed green beans.

Vegan Thai Coconut Curry (p184)
Coconut milk broth, combined with chickpeas, bell peppers, aromatic red curry paste, spicy ginger, and sweet mango.

Pork Chops with Sweet Cinnamon Apples (p192)
Savory pork chops with a sweet brown sugar rub and warm cinnamon apples, paired with tender sweet potatoes.

Italian Stuffed Bell Peppers
Baked bell peppers stuffed with white beans, cherry tomatoes, zucchini, onions, and farro, seasoned with Italian seasoning and topped with fresh basil.

<u>Pesto and Roasted Veggie Pasta</u> (p178)
Lentil pasta, broccoli, and zucchini, combined with a
homemade pesto made with olive oil, pine nuts, parmesan
cheese, zippy lemon, and sweet basil.

<u>Slow Cooker Pot Roast</u>
Beef round, Yukon gold potatoes, baby carrots, and sliced
onions, made in a slow cooker.

<u>Blended Carrot Ginger Soup</u> (p168)
Vibrant turmeric and ginger, rich and creamy coconut milk,
roasted carrots and sweet potatoes, topped with crispy
chickpeas.

<u>Chicken Tenders</u>
Baked chicken tenders, corn on the cob, and coleslaw made
with yogurt, vinegar, and lemon juice.

Snacks

Baked cinnamon apple chips.

Medjool date stuffed with unsalted peanut butter.

Celery sticks with nut butter.

Corn chips with low-sodium salsa.

Roasted chickpeas with smoked paprika and cumin.

Strawberries and assorted berries chopped into plain, nonfat Greek yogurt.

Plain popcorn with homemade parmesan garlic or smoky BBQ seasoning.

Fruit skewers with low-fat cheese cubes, strawberries, and grapes.

Homemade trail mix with sunflower seeds, pepitas, dried cranberries, and raisins.

Hummus topped cucumber bites.

Steamed artichoke with lemon pepper dip.

Bell pepper strips with guacamole.

Roasted carrots with carrot-top pesto.

Hard-boiled egg with your choice of pesto, low-sodium mustard, or guacamole.

Nut butter covered banana bites.

Your choice of sliced fruit and unsalted nuts.

CHAPTER SEVEN

Supercharge Your Weight Loss

Like a broken record, we hear all the time that weight loss is good for a long healthy life. But why exactly? You'd be surprised to know that there is a good correlation between weight loss and blood pressure. Research that looked at weight loss in overweight and obese individuals found improvements in their blood pressure readings as well as in their lab values related to heart disease. Losing just 5% of their body weight within one to three years reduced systolic blood pressure by 3 mm Hg and diastolic blood pressure by 2 mm Hg.[50] [51] Those who kept the weight off improved their blood pressure readings even further.

If you are working on improving your cholesterol or triglycerides, we have more good news for you. Research found that losing 6.6 pounds averaged a drop of 15 mg/dL in triglycerides, while losing anywhere from 11 to 17.6 pounds reduced LDL-C (your "bad" cholesterol) by 5 mg/dL and improved HDL-C (your "good" cholesterol") by 2-3 mg/dL.[52] [53] From this information, you may find motivation knowing that weight loss can help lower your blood pressure, while also benefiting your cholesterol and triglyceride levels. Even if you don't have elevated cholesterol or triglyceride labs, weight loss is a good preventative measure.

Setting Goals

In general, weight loss of no more than one to two pounds per week is the ideal amount to lose weight slowly and sustainably. Remember, we want to lose just enough to be able to maintain the weight loss for the rest of our life. Nice and slow is the name of the game! Losing one pound a week will result in a 52-pound weight loss in one year, which is a lot! Even if you lose one-half of a pound per week, you will be down 26 pounds in 12 months. If you have struggled with losing weight, you know 26 pounds is a difficult accomplishment.

No matter how much weight you lose (or gain or maintain) in a week, never get discouraged. Keep going! Life is not perfect, and your weight loss journey will not be perfect either. Instead of telling yourself, "I only lost half a pound this week," change your mentality to, "I lost half a pound. That's a great achievement, and I can't wait to see my progress next week!". The most important part about weight loss is consistency. Stick to your diet and exercise, and you will see results.

Let's have a look at calculating your own personalized weight loss target. The recommended amount of weight loss for better health and to help lower your blood pressure is 5 to 10% weight loss in the first six months. Calculate your weight loss goal by multiplying your current weight by 0.05 and 0.10 to get your weight loss range. Therefore, if you weigh 180 pounds, multiply 180 pounds by 0.05 and 0.10. The weight loss goal will be 9 to 18 pounds in six months. You can also calculate how much weight you need to lose weekly. There are 24 weeks in 6 months, so divide both numbers by 24 to get the amount of weight loss you should lose every week to reach your goal in 6 months. If you weigh 180 pounds and your weight loss range is between 9 to 18 pounds in six months, you need to lose about 3/4 of a pound a week to reach your goal. It sounds doable when you calculate it this way, right?

The Recipe for Success

While weight loss is not the definitive goal in DASH, incorporating the DASH food groups into your regimen, and following our recommended serving guidelines which have been specifically tailored for weight loss, can undoubtedly result in lower numbers on the scale. But what can you do to give your weight loss efforts that boost to ensure you are seeing the results you desire?

Is there a recipe for weight loss success? Technically, yes! An observational study that spanned over ten years studied individuals who successfully lost weight and maintained it. Participants were asked to list the factors that they feel helped them the most to lose the weight and keep it off. The study concluded that the biggest contributing factors to their weight loss were following a suitable diet, incorporating exercise, monitoring their food intake, reducing emotional eating, and never skipping meals.[54]

We've got you covered on the first factor on the list. The DASH diet is your best diet of choice for reducing blood pressure and losing weight. Let's look at the remaining factors to determine if and how you can incorporate them into your daily life.

Physical Activity

Moving more will help you shed more pounds, but how much more do you need to move? With physical activity, we want to slowly and gently move into a physically active lifestyle. Jumping right into something like CrossFit tomorrow will cause overexertion and muscle injuries, which will physically hold you back on your progress.

Let's evaluate your current physical activity. Go through a typical day in your head. How much time do you spend sleeping, watching TV, walking, standing, and driving? Does your regular day consist of other activities such as hiking, swimming, or climbing stairs? Write these down on a piece of paper, along with the hours or minutes you think you spend on each activity during a regular day. How many minutes a day would you say you are active? The results may surprise you. A general guideline is 30 minutes a day, or at least 150 minutes a week.

If you find that you are physically inactive most of the day, start identifying times when you can squeeze in an activity. If you live in a walking-friendly area, go for a walk around the block after dinner. If you have a gym membership, download your favorite show and watch it while you take a few laps on the treadmill. Rather take the stairs up one floor instead of taking the elevator. These are just a few ideas, but the key is to slowly start incorporating physical activity in a way that works for you, your schedule, and your fitness level.

Also, decide what types of exercise or physical activity you enjoy! If you enjoy it, you are more likely to do it more often and be able to keep it up. You might prefer doing exercises in the privacy of your home, like online dance and conditioning classes, bodyweight workouts, jump rope, roughhousing with your kids, or simply walking around in your apartment while listening to a podcast. Or you might prefer working out outdoors, like bike riding, hiking, swimming, taking up a sport such as golf or tennis, or just going for a walk to the store if you live or work nearby.

When you're starting out, 150 minutes of activity is recommended per week at a moderate-intensity level. "Moderate-intensity" can be described as enough to get your heart rate up to where speaking takes a little more effort, but you are still able to carry on a conversation without gasping for air. Once you decide you are ready for more intense exercise, you can change to 75 minutes of activity at a vigorous-intensity level. "Vigorous-intensity" is characterized by a substantially higher heart rate and rapid breathing, to where you can speak only a few words at a time and not in full sentences.[55]

One last tip is to invest in a pedometer or fitness tracker. There are quite inexpensive options on the market, and they are terrific tools to help you track your activity levels throughout the day.

Counting Calories

Counting calories and macros (protein, carbs, and fat) is a subject that has been blown out of proportion recently. Some say it's the best way to control your intake to lose weight, while others say it's a borderline eating disorder. The question most people have when they start on their nutrition journey is: "Should I count calories?" The simple answer is "No", and we'll explain why.

First, what do we mean by counting calories? All foods are broken down into energy and have a caloric value based on how much protein, carbs, and fat are in them. Our bodies need a certain number of calories to function daily. On a basic level, if you eat more than this number you will gain weight, and if you eat less than this number you will lose weight. Counting calories refers to the act of logging the calories contained in each meal you eat, to hit a predetermined calorie target in a day.

Logging calories and macros is an effective way to manage your weight, but it comes with some drawbacks. The biggest of which is it being a time-consuming and somewhat complicated method. It requires you to determine how many calories your body needs, to choose an appropriate macro-split, and then to track how many calories and macros you eat every day. This is completely unnecessary on a diet such as DASH, which promotes nutritious foods, provides guidelines in terms of serving sizes, and has recommended daily servings tailored for weight loss.

A handy tool we do recommend is keeping a food diary. Write down what you ate, as well as the number of servings. You can also specify if something is whole wheat, which part of the chicken you ate, and if it was skinless or not, and include the type of oil you used when cooking. This is completely optional, but a food diary will allow you to compare your daily meals to the DASH guidelines, and eventually make adjustments to your diet to suit your preferences.

Mindful Eating

Mindless eating happens when you eat even when you are not hungry. This can happen when you feel bored, stressed, emotional, or watching a movie. Mindless eating is unconscious and automatic, where you eat without enjoying or remembering the food. This kind of consumption can go on for years and results in overeating, excessive calorie intake, and weight gain.[56] By incorporating principles of mindful eating, it can help you identify times when you may be tempted to eat mindlessly versus eating for hunger or enjoyment. Being mindfully aware allows you to figure out what triggers can cause mindless eating. This awareness is what will allow you to change your actions.

Based on the research, practicing mindful eating can improve stress levels in people with depression and chronic pain, it can lower blood sugar levels in patients with type 2 diabetes, it can reduce binge eating by over 60%, and it can improve weight loss efforts for those who struggle with their weight.[56] When applied to DASH, mindful eating can be a simple and effective tool you can incorporate to prevent overeating and help improve your overall eating behaviors.

Incorporating mindful eating takes conscious effort at the beginning but can become second nature over time. Mindful eating is not about restriction but about identifying triggers that can cause overeating or eating beyond your hunger and fullness cues. In the Eat What You Love, Love What You Eat book from Michelle May, she goes through a series of questions that can help you identify these triggers.[57]

❀ **Why do you eat?**

Are you eating because of stress? Are you grabbing food because you had a bad day at work? Do you turn to food after an argument or whenever you receive bad news? Are you bored and trying to keep yourself busy by eating? Once you start figuring out why you eat, you may find that there are times in your life when you are eating without actually being hungry.

❀ **When do you eat?**

Do you always feel like you need a snack when you're catching up on your favorite show? Are you skipping breakfast or lunch and only making do with snacks? Observing when you eat is something to consider to help you eat more mindfully.

❀ **What do you eat?**

Are you grabbing fast and convenient food when you're on the go or after a long day at work? Are you eating nutritious meals for breakfast? Being aware of what you eat plays a big role in the DASH diet.

❀ **How do you eat?**

Are you eating in a rush at your desk at work? Are you eating while distracted by social media on your phone? How you are eating is an area you can work on by slowing down to enjoy your food or turning off your phone before you eat.

❀ **How much do you eat?**

Are you eating even after feeling full? When you grab a bag of snacks, do you eat the entire bag? Do you eat the last few bites because you are still hungry, or is it an unconscious habit to clean the plate? Identifying these habits can help you make changes to habitually eating less.

Asking these questions every day will help you increase your awareness of your eating behaviors and habits. This is not a tool to judge you or make you feel bad for eating. When you can slow down to appreciate all the flavors, textures, and aromas in your food, you will find that eating is enjoyable! Slowing down also gives you time to figure out your hunger and fullness cues. Mindful eating will take some practice, but the proven health benefits will be incredible in your DASH journey!

CHAPTER EIGHT

Staying on Track

In the previous chapter, we looked at setting realistic goals for weight loss, as well as the success factors that will take your weight loss to the next level. We also discussed keeping a food diary to keep track of your daily meals and the foods you eat. In this chapter, we'll have a look at a few basic metrics you can use to track your weight loss progress over time. A food diary should ideally be tracked daily, while the metrics we will discuss here can be tracked as often as you like, although once a week is recommended.

Throughout this journey, remember that losing weight slowly is the best method for maintaining weight loss over time. Losing a mass amount of weight in a short period will cause your body to do everything in its ability to regain the weight. Eating more fruits and vegetables and going for more walks is much more sustainable for your body than eliminating carbohydrates or going on a juice cleanse for two weeks.

Tracking Your Weight Loss

The humble bathroom scale is most people's first port of call when it comes to tracking their weight loss. But your weight is only one part of your progress and doesn't give the entire picture of what is going on in your body. Your body composition can change significantly, while the numbers on the scale remain more or less the same. This is especially true if you start to work out more. It's like comparing two houses with the same square footage. One might be a modern dream home, while the other requires a complete remodel. Let's look at a few popular methods for measuring and tracking your weight loss.

Body Mass Index

Using BMI as a determining factor for weight loss is a controversial issue. The measurement only looks at height and weight and has no indication of an individual's body composition, such as body fat percentage.[58] An extreme example as to why BMI is not a good indicator of being overweight or obese is with athletes and bodybuilders. This group tends to be heavy on the scale while having very little body fat. Therefore, their BMI indicates they are overweight, while their body fat percentage can be in the single digits. We still feel it's worthwhile mentioning BMI because it is quick, inexpensive, and convenient to do at home. The formula for measuring your body mass index is shown below.

$$BMI = \frac{\text{weight in kilograms}}{\text{height in meters}^2} \qquad \begin{aligned} kg &= lbs \div 2.2 \\ m &= in \times 0.0254 \end{aligned}$$

As you may have noticed, the equation uses metric units. But we can easily convert imperial to metric with a bit of math. To get kilograms, divide your weight in pounds by 2.2, and to get meters, multiply your height in inches by 0.0254. It's important to note that height is squared in the equation.

Let's look at an example by calculating the BMI of someone who is 5'4" and weighs 180 pounds. Converting these measurements to metric units, we get 1.6256 meters and 81.82 kilograms. Since the equation asks for height squared, we can use a calculator or multiply 1.6256 by 1.6256 to get 2.6426. Finally, we complete the calculation by dividing 81.82 by 2.6426 to get 30.96. We can then compare this number to the rages provided by the Centers for Disease Control and Prevention which classifies 30.96 as obese.[59]

CDC BMI categories

BMI	*Weight Status*
Below 18.5	Underweight
18.5 - 24.9	Healthy Weight
25.0 - 29.9	Overweight
30.0 and above	Obese

Go ahead and calculate your BMI right now. No matter what category you get, do not let it get you down! This is simply a measurement you can track over time as you embark on your DASH journey, not a label you should use to classify your weight.

Waist Circumference

Waist circumference is a measurement used to measure body fat distribution. Clinically, fat distribution is classified in two ways: central (or abdominal) and lower body.[55] Central body fat distribution refers to where most of the fat is stored around the waist and the abdominal organs. This type of body shape is known as an "apple" shape and is more commonly seen in men.[55] Lower body fat distribution refers to where most of the fat is stored around the hips and thighs, known as a "pear" shape and more commonly seen in women.[55]

Between the two types of distributions, the central body fat type is paired with risks of type 2 diabetes, dyslipidemia, hypertension, and coronary heart disease. On the other hand, the lower body fat type does not carry the same risks and, in some studies, has shown a negative correlation to both diabetes and cardiovascular disease.[60 61]

There are a few ways to measure the amount of fat in both distribution types, the most accurate methods are magnetic resonance imaging (MRI) and computed tomography (CT) scans. Unfortunately, these techniques are expensive and not easily accessible for most. Instead, we can measure our waist circumference, which is an alternative method that is cheap and much easier to do! Results are comparable to an MRI or CT scan as a risk indicator for cardiovascular disease.[55] The only tool you will need is a flexible measuring tape!

To get your waist circumference, simply measure horizontally around your waist at the belly button level. Relax your abdomen (do not suck it in), and rest the tape measure comfortably around your waist. Do not squeeze your waist tightly with the measuring tape. If you're a man with a waist circumference greater than 40 inches or a woman with a circumference greater than 35 inches, you are at risk for cardiovascular diseases, diabetes, and hypertension.[62]

If you fall under the lower body fat category, it's also recommended to measure the circumference around your hip. To measure your hip, wrap the tape measure around the widest part of your hip and buttocks. As a reminder, do not wrap the measuring tape too tightly. Waist and hip circumference are measurements you can track throughout your DASH journey, and are numbers you can see decrease as you change your diet and move more.

With both your waist and hip measurements you can calculate your waist-to-hip ratio (WHR). This is done by dividing your waist circumference by your hip circumference. The result will only be greater than 1.0 if your waist circumference is higher than your hip circumference. In terms of risk indications, the determining factor is different between men and women. Men with a WHR greater than 1.0 and women with a WHR greater than 0.8 are at increased risk for health problems.[63]

Advanced Techniques

Other than calculating your body mass index and measuring your waist and hip circumference, there are more advanced techniques available to determine your body composition. One such method involves skinfold measurements, where they pinch your skin on various parts of your body to measure body fat using a caliper. This test is widely available at many health clubs and is usually not too expensive. Something to note is that the results are very dependent on the person giving you the test, how experienced they are, and the quality of the calipers they use. It is quite difficult to grab fat consistently to measure with a caliper, so results can vary significantly.[64]

Recently, some bathroom scales have started to incorporate bioelectrical impedance analysis (BIA) to measure body fat. BIA sends small electrical impulses through your body and measures the resistance it encounters from the different tissues. These numbers are plugged into an equation to then determine your body fat percentage. Unfortunately, body fat scales are not very accurate when compared to lab-based tests and can read up to 8% higher or lower.[65] The readings are also affected by many factors such as time of day, fluid intake, and the type of training you do. However, all things considered, they are an easy way to keep track of your weight loss at home.

If you are looking for the most accurate readings available, you can go to specialized centers or research labs at universities for ultra-advanced methods such as dual-energy X-ray absorptiometry (DEXA) scans, underwater weighing, and air-displacement plethysmography. Some of these tests can get quite expensive. If you are considering one of these methods, we recommend speaking to your physician for recommendations in your area.

Tracking your measurements is a great way to measure your progress as you lose weight and lower your blood pressure. Of course, tracking these numbers are up to you. Keep in mind that not monitoring your measurements can make it hard to see your progress in the short term. If we look at ourselves in the mirror every day, we usually don't notice the small changes that are happening to our bodies. Tracking makes the results undeniable, and your path to better health should be celebrated along the way!

Hitting a Plateau

After the first six months of weight loss, you might experience a plateau, where additional weight loss becomes exceptionally more difficult.[66] There doesn't seem to be a consensus on why this happens. Many theorize that your body simply adapts to the weight loss or slows down metabolism due to the weight loss. Researchers studying weight loss plateaus concluded that these theories do not hold enough merit and that the likely reason for weight loss plateaus are that people simply don't stick to their diets and exercise plans.[66]

Whatever the reason, it is important to not be hard on yourself during this time. Keep eating nutritious foods, make time for physical activity, and your body will soon adjust to weight loss again. Do not give up! This might be a great time to make some adjustments to your meals and workouts. Go through the DASH foods list to see if there are foods you haven't tried before, and look for delicious recipes you can use them in. Change up your exercise routine by trying a new outdoor activity. Making a few small changes can reinvigorate your drive and jumpstart the weight loss machine.

What's Next?

Everyone's weight loss journey will be different. You have been given a lot of information and tools to help you lose weight on the DASH diet. Take your time in this chapter and the previous chapter, as you take your measurements, interpret your data, and set goals. Remember to find your motivation by looking back at the why you have written down at the beginning of the book. You may come back to these chapters often while you make your lifestyle changes.

In the upcoming chapters, we will explore the research behind the DASH diet and have a closer look at the factors that lead to hypertension. We will show you how to read nutrition labels in finding DASH-friendly foods. Then we will help you get started in the kitchen if you are a novice chef, before diving into 30 delicious recipes for every meal of the day.

What have you tried so far?

If you found any part of this guide helpful up until now, or learned something new that you can't wait to try out, I would love to hear about it. The main way for me to connect with you is through a review on Amazon. So head over there and let me know which topics you liked most, or even which ones you didn't like. Have you started to apply any of the advice in this guide? I would love to hear about it as well.

CHAPTER NINE

Getting Nerdy with DASH

In the following few chapters, put on your science hat because we will delve into the research that has led to DASH being the number one diet for hypertension, we will have a closer look at the ins and outs of blood pressure and how it works, as well as going deeper into hypertension, what causes it, and the potential health risks if high blood pressure is not managed. There is no better way to understand hypertension than to learn how your body works and how the decisions you make affect it. In this chapter, we'll start by looking at the clinical trials that have been conducted on the DASH diet.

The trials were sparked by researchers recognizing that vegetarians tend to have better blood pressure than non-vegetarians. This led to the hypothesis that vegetarians may have excellent blood pressure due to a higher intake of specific micronutrients such as magnesium and potassium. Studies tested purely supplementing with these nutrients and found little effect on blood pressure.[12] The problem was, the body may not register supplements as well as naturally occurring nutrients in foods. It was also possible that blood pressure responds better to all of the nutrients together through a wholesome diet.[12] Therefore, the following trials were conducted to test this theory.

DASH Trial

The DASH trial was the first clinical study backed by the National Heart, Lung, and Blood Institute (NHLBI). It was conducted by scientists from major schools and universities in the United States. The trial focused on finding the nutritional effects on blood pressure using an eating plan that had the right number of fruits and vegetables and other foods low in cholesterol and saturated fats.[67]

459 adults participated in the study, with 133 of them having high blood pressure over 140/90 mm Hg.[12] None of the subjects were taking any blood pressure medication, vitamins, or supplements. Participants were randomly assigned either a typical American diet (high in saturated fat and cholesterol) with increased fruits and vegetables and fewer sweets, or the DASH diet which included low-fat dairy as well as foods low in saturated fats and high in protein and fiber. They were on this diet for eight weeks, and each diet contained 3,000 milligrams of sodium per day.

At the end of the trial, the results showed that blood pressure was lowered in both diets compared to the control diet, but those who were on DASH had the best results.[67] Even participants who had normal blood pressure saw a reduction of 2.8 mm Hg in their systolic number and a 1.1 mm Hg reduction in their diastolic reading after being on the DASH diet.

For those who had high blood pressure, their blood pressure was reduced by 11.1 mm Hg (systolic) and by 5.5 mm Hg in their diastolic.[12] A reduction in blood pressure was already observed during the first two weeks and maintained for the duration of the trial. After the trial was conducted, follow-up reports found that the DASH diet also helped lower cholesterol.[3]

Since blood pressure lowered even for those who had normal blood pressure, the results indicate that adopting the DASH diet can be essential to preventing potential hypertension. Subjects who were hypertensive had even more remarkable results in their readings. The results were comparable to those found in trials using antihypertensive medication! Therefore, DASH can be seen as a nutrition alternative to preventing and improving hypertension without the use of drugs. Scientists also concluded that if the majority of Americans adopted the DASH diet, stroke occurrences could reduce by 27% and coronary heart disease by 15%. That is a big deal!

DASH-Sodium Trial

The DASH-Sodium trial was the second study published and was conducted by the same scientists who undertook the initial DASH trial. They wanted to take another step forward into the effects of DASH. From the first DASH trial, we know that increasing fruits and vegetables lowered blood pressure, even with 3,000 mg of sodium per day. As of the late 1990s, clinical trials were publishing the positive correlation between low-sodium diets and blood pressure.[10] Based on this data, national guidelines started encouraging U.S. citizens to consume less than 2,300 mg of sodium per day.

The research team decided to test this low-sodium idea by applying it to both a typical American diet and to the DASH diet. They also wanted to test an even lower sodium diet of 1,500 mg, 35% less than the daily recommendation. The trial had 412 total participants of which 41% were hypertensive. Three sodium levels were tested for each diet: 3,300 mg, 2,400 mg, and 1,500 mg. Whenever the sodium levels were decreased, blood pressure also reduced on each diet plan, with those who were on the DASH diet seeing the most notable reduction.[67]

For the hypertensive participants, systolic blood pressure on the low-sodium DASH diet resulted in a decrease of 11.5 mm Hg in systolic blood pressure while the non-hypertensive dropped by 7.1 mm Hg. Women also saw a larger systolic reduction of 10.5 mm Hg while the men fell by 6.8 mm Hg.[10] After the

DASH-Sodium trial, the researchers were able to confidently say that pairing the recommended low-sodium intake with the DASH diet had the best results in lowering blood pressure and treating hypertension.[10]

OmniHeart Trial

The first two trials we looked at were conducted in the 1990s. Now let's move forward into the next decade: the 2000s. During this time, specific fad diets were gaining popularity in the United States. People were trying out the low-carb South Beach diet or the high-protein Atkins diet. These diets were truly trendy at the time and, although you don't hear about them nowadays, you hear or see them in various forms such as the Keto and Paleo diets.

Based on these trends, researchers wanted to test a few variations of the DASH diet to see if they lowered blood pressure, serum lipids, and decreased estimated cardiovascular risk. This third trial, termed OmniHeart (short for Optimal Macronutrient Intake Trial to Prevent Heart Disease), included a total of 164 participants, all with either prehypertension or hypertension. None of the participants were on antihypertensive medication, and the trial lasted 19 weeks.

The entire study was designed to mimic a regular DASH diet with two additional lower-carb variations. One replaced 10% of carbohydrates with protein. The majority of the increased protein was plant-based, with a slight increase in animal-based protein. The second variation replaced 10% of carbohydrates with unsaturated fats. These extra fats came from olive oil spreads, and olive and canola oils. Other than the above changes, all diets followed the DASH guidelines and limited sodium to 2,300 mg per day.

All three diets had positive effects in lowering blood pressure, total cholesterol, LDL levels, and reducing the risk of cardiovascular disease by 16% to 21%.[68] Although results were best when 10% of daily carbohydrates were replaced with either protein or unsaturated fat sources.[68] There is an assumption that cutting carbs is healthy, but the OmniHeart trial supports the idea that incorporating a healthy amount of carbohydrates in your diet can still aid in your goals for lowering blood pressure. If you decide to cut carbs, cutting just 10% and replacing it with plant-based proteins or heart-healthy fats can have additional benefits of lowering triglycerides.

OmniCarb Trial

We will keep the OmniCarb trial short as the setup is very similar to the other DASH trials. It was published in 2014 and focused on the effects of carbohydrates on cardiovascular disease and diabetes. The researchers wanted to determine if individuals on the DASH diet needed to concern themselves with the glycemic index or GI of carbohydrates. If you have never heard of the glycemic index before, it assigns a number to specific carb-rich foods to indicate how fast it raises your blood glucose. A carbohydrate with a low GI, such as oats, whole wheat bread, and beans, does not spike your blood sugar as fast as a carbohydrate with a high GI, such as potatoes, white bread, and macaroni.[69]

Scientists tested a variation of high and low glycemic carbs. They concluded that selecting foods low on the glycemic index while combined with the DASH diet, did not improve blood pressure or lipid levels in their participants. Therefore, they were not able to support the idea that low glycemic carbs can reduce the risk of cardiovascular disease.[70] It is however worthwhile to note that it has been found that low GI foods will keep you fuller for longer, compared to high GI foods.[71]

An earlier study done in 2004 of over 2000 individuals spanning 5 years concluded that GI did have a negative effect on insulin sensitivity and insulin resistance.[72] So if you are sensitive to carbohydrates or have diabetes, it might be worthwhile to aim for low GI foods. The two main factors that determine GI are fiber and complexity. These characteristics are rarely present in processed foods, so aiming for natural unprocessed foods would be more than enough if you do not fall in this group.

Premier Trial

If you're looking at losing weight while on DASH, then the Premier trial is worth taking note of. Up to this point, the other DASH trials were focused on food and nutrition while keeping lifestyle factors constant. The Premier trial wanted to focus on whether or not blood pressure could be reduced if individuals were put on a program that encouraged lifestyle changes, such as physical activity. The trial had a total of 810 participants who all had blood pressure higher than 120/80 mm Hg. None of them were on blood pressure medication and most were physically inactive and overweight.

The participants were divided into one of three different groups for six months. The first group only received a 30-minute session with a Registered Dietitian for advice on blood pressure. The second group incorporated physical activity for 180 minutes per week and reduced sodium intake to 2,400 mg per day. The third group was required to do everything the second group did but was also placed on the DASH diet for the duration of the trial.

Blood pressure dropped for participants in all three groups, but those who were in the DASH group saw the most significant decrease of 14.2 mm Hg (systolic) and 7.4 mm Hg (diastolic).[73] This group also experienced the most significant weight loss. Because blood pressure was lowered in all three programs, it means that having some nutrition education and background on how blood pressure works can steer you in the right direction. If you tack on physical activity, DASH guidelines, and eating just a little fewer calories, you are on your way to dropping both your blood pressure and those pounds!

The recommendations in this book are based on these trials and similar research, to provide you with the best possible solution to lower not only your blood pressure but also your weight. Most of the participants had high blood pressure, some were overweight, most had a sedentary lifestyle, and they were able to lower their blood pressure and weight while reducing their risk of cardiovascular disease by following the DASH diet and getting more active. These studies also included participants from all different socioeconomic backgrounds, genders, and ethnicities and found a positive impact in all groups.

CHAPTER TEN

Blood Pressure & Hypertension

In this section, we'll be looking at the physiology of blood pressure. Understanding how our cardiovascular system works allows us to understand how the decisions we make impact our health. This basic understanding of blood pressure provides the background needed to get a grip on why hypertension occurs. We will also learn how our bodies regulate blood pressure, how blood pressure medications work, and different classifications of hypertension. Then we will dive into the various factors that can lead to hypertension, helping you to avoid them in your own life.

How Your Body Regulates Blood Pressure

In addition to delivering oxygen and nutrients throughout our bodies,[74] our cardiovascular system also works in maintaining and regulating our fluids, body temperature, hormones, pH levels, and the exchange of gases.[55] Blood pressure is the force of blood on the walls of our blood vessels as our hearts pump blood through our blood vessels, arteries, and capillaries to perform these functions.[18] The speed of our blood flow depends on how much nutrition our bodies need. For example, if you are exercising vigorously, your muscles need more oxygen and nutrients. Your heart can then increase blood flow by three- to fourfold to meet your body's needs.[75]

Aside from survival, our bodies' other main goal is equilibrium. Our blood pressure changes slightly throughout the day. For example, when we get out of bed in the morning, it tends to spike but is quickly balanced by our baroreceptor reflex.[76] The baroreceptors are useful for quick fixes, and without them, we would feel dizzy every time our blood pressure changes. In times of stress, our so-called "fight or flight" response triggers a different system. In an emergency, our nervous system temporarily closes the baroreceptors and turns on the Renin-Angiotensin-Aldosterone System, or RAAS for short.

When RAAS is triggered a few hormones are called to action: Renin, Angiotensin, and Aldosterone (hence the name RAAS). These hormones are released by the body to signal your kidneys to retain water and sodium. By doing this, the body can increase blood volume to create more flow. Hormones will also communicate with your blood vessels to contract harder. All of this increases blood pressure. When your blood pressure is low again, RAAS is turned off by releasing the first hormone: Renin.[76] Your body has many parameters and signals in place to keep your blood pressure as steady as possible. It is complicated but quite amazing!

So now we understand how our bodies maintain blood pressure using baroreceptor reflexes for small changes and RAAS in urgent situations. While these systems are set in place to keep us balanced and alive, RAAS is not supposed to be used often. Unfortunately, having hypertension enforces RAAS frequently and inappropriately. Aside from hypertension, RAAS can also be activated in cases of heart failure, diabetes, and acute heart attacks.[76] The increased pressure in hypertension can wear out your blood vessels and organs, and lead to further complications. Therefore, it's essential to treat hypertension as soon as possible.

How Blood Pressure Medications Work

Whether you are currently taking blood pressure medication, or your doctor has suggested getting you on one, this section will help you understand how each type of medication works. A common type of medication you might have heard of is loop diuretics, also known as a "water pill". In the pharmaceutical world, they go by the names of furosemide, torsemide, or bumetanide, and are used to flush your system of water and sodium.[77] With less water in your blood vessels, there is less blood volume, therefore lower blood pressure. Sodium is also flushed out since it retains water in your body.

Another conventional medication is an ACE inhibitor. ACE is the enzyme that converts angiotensin I to angiotensin II so angiotensin II can signal your body to increase blood pressure. These ACE inhibitors do precisely as the name implies, it inhibits the ACE enzyme. Without angiotensin II, your body cannot increase blood pressure. Other names for the ACE inhibitor medications include lisinopril, enalapril, and captopril.[78]

Drugs called propranolol, acebutolol, and atenolol are beta-adrenergic blocking agents. These medications block the heart's beta-receptors, which get activated by stress hormones. By blocking these receptors, the stress hormones cannot bind to them, therefore preventing an increase in blood pressure.[79] Similarly, alpha-receptor antagonists is another set of medication that makes the heart muscles ignore stress hormones. In return, the volume of blood pumped from the heart is reduced, resulting in lowered pressure.[79] These drugs also go by the names terazosin, doxazosin, and prazosin.

When you hear of calcium, you probably think of it as a nutrient you find in milk and how it helps build strong bones. But calcium also acts as an electrolyte to contract your muscles. Calcium channel-blocking agents, also called verapamil, blocks some of these calcium channels. This mechanism prevents the entrance of calcium into the muscle tissues, allowing your blood vessels to relax and contract less.[55] Lastly, we have aldosterone antagonists, called either spironolactone or eplerenone. These medications prevent aldosterone from working, which if you recall, is a component of RAAS. By keeping aldosterone at bay, it becomes another mechanism to keep your blood pressure managed.[55]

High Blood Pressure Classifications

Did you know there are various classifications for blood pressure? The American Heart Association groups blood pressure into the five categories depicted in the chart below.[80] If your levels ever exceed a systolic pressure of 180 mm Hg and/or a diastolic pressure of 120 mm Hg, it is crucial to contact your doctor's office. This level can indicate urgent health concerns such as a stroke or heart attack.[81] Increased blood pressure can also affect your vision and kidney health. If your blood pressure reaches this crisis level, and it is paired with nosebleeds, shortness of breath, anxiety, or headaches, call the emergency services immediately.

As you start making lifestyle changes while following this guide, and you track the progress of your blood pressure, compare your numbers to the chart above to see if your blood pressure level changes. Ideally, we would like to see it get into the normal range. If you are diagnosed with hypertension or prescribed antihypertensive medications, you are still considered at risk of hypertension, even if you can keep and maintain it at a normal range. At this point, maintenance will be key!

AHA blood pressure categories

Category	Systolic (upper number)	Diastolic (lower number)
Normal	Less than 120	Less than 80
Elevated	120 - 129	Less than 80
High (Hypertension Stage 1)	130 - 139	80 - 89
High (Hypertension Stage 2)	140 - 179	90 - 119
Hypertensive Crisis	180 or higher	120 or higher

Risk Factors for Hypertension

Getting diagnosed with hypertension can leave you with feelings of confusion, causing you to ask yourself, "Why?". Perhaps you have family members who also have high blood pressure and concluded that the problem is genetic. Or maybe you thought about sodium and started looking at reducing your salt intake. In this section, we'll review the multiple risk factors for hypertension. As you go through them, compare them to your current situation to see if they apply to you. This will also help you to determine if any lifestyle changes are needed.

When looking at these risk factors, keep in mind that there are two ways to classify hypertension: primary and secondary.[74] Around 90 to 95 percent of cases are classified as primary hypertension, also known as essential hypertension.[74] You are diagnosed with primary hypertension if the cause is unknown. While research suggests there are various risk factors causing high blood pressure, it is difficult to pinpoint the exact origin of someone's hypertension. It can range from lack of physical activity to stress to an overactive RAAS system. It can even be a combination of factors.

The second classification is secondary hypertension, meaning hypertension is the secondary condition, caused by another significant condition. For example, hypertension can result from kidney or cardiovascular diseases, or disorders of the endocrine and nervous systems.[55] This classification is more specific and can be quickly narrowed down by your doctor based on specific conditions. Since most cases are primary hypertension, we will review risk factors for this classification in greater detail.

Stress

Stress is essential to understand since it affects your body's nervous system. It is an underlying problem for many diseases and health conditions, and it can trigger specific hormones that can cause your blood vessels and organs to stay overactive.[82] If stress is not managed, it can result in chronic hypertension. Stress causes your body to act abnormally. Certain conditions like obesity can cause your body to be under stress internally, whether or not you realize it. Stress affects our autonomic nervous system, which is the involuntary nervous system our bodies have in place. This system works autonomously and regulates our gastrointestinal activities, blood pressure, bladder, eyes, and body heat.[82]

Imagine you are attending an annual company meeting. You sit in the audience with a few of your close co-workers while eating a couple of items from the catered lunch. With everything set, you find yourself laughing with your team and preparing for the next couple of hours to be fun and relaxing. Thirty minutes into the meeting, all is well. Your boss is called to the stage to discuss your team's success.

She gives you credit for securing the most prominent client. You smile and wave as everyone in the audience turns around to look at you. Then, all of a sudden, she asks you to come up to make a speech. Your boss never told you she would do this, so you came unprepared. Left with no choice, you awkwardly walk to the stage to stand behind the podium. Everyone is staring at you, waiting for you to say something. You start breathing heavily, eyes become wide open, your stomach twists into a knot, and your hands become sweaty. Your heart is racing at what feels like 100 miles an hour.

This is our autonomic nervous system, or more specifically our sympathetic nervous system, which is triggered in times of stress or danger.[82] Many circumstances can trigger stress like taking an exam, impressing someone on a first date, or dreading the results of your recent blood work. You will get similar stress responses regardless of which situation you are dealing with. Your body only knows one thing: you are stressed, and it needs to survive. If you are always stressed from work or life, you are unconsciously triggering your blood pressure to rise. Getting stress under control is an integral part of lowering and maintaining blood pressure.

Find therapeutic activities to help you destress, whether it is reading or hiking, and make it a time for self-care. If appropriate, seek professional help for stress management. Aside from hypertension, stress can also be a contributor to weight gain. Stress releases a hormone called cortisol, which triggers your appetite and leads to unintentional overeating.[83] This reason is another motivation to manage stress as it can make it difficult for you to achieve your weight loss goals.

Obesity

Obesity is a national issue and a risk factor for hypertension. The more weight you gain, the more strain on your heart, cardiovascular system, and lungs.[55] Another risk factor for high blood pressure is excess body fat stored around your waist and stomach.[18] The effect of this additional weight can be seen when looking at any cardio activity, such as jogging. Losing just 10 pounds can significantly reduce the workload on your cardiorespiratory system, increasing your functional capacity to perform the exercise. In other words, you can jog longer or faster with the same amount of effort.

This explanation is a simplified one. More specifically, there are physiological explanations as to how being overweight or obese can cause hypertension. The first is that the additional weight requires additional blood flow to the muscles, kidneys, heart, and gastrointestinal tract, to compensate for the extra fat tissue, increased metabolism, and growth of organs and tissues that come with weight gain.[74] This extra blood flow leads to an increase in vascular resistance over time, resulting in chronic hypertension.[84]

Another reason for how excess weight can cause chronic high blood pressure is an overactive sympathetic nervous system affecting the kidneys. Researchers have found this characteristic in overweight patients and believe leptin, a hormone released by fat cells, may excite the hypothalamus which can overstimulate the sympathetic nervous system. This can impair kidney function, requiring an increase in blood pressure for the kidneys to function normally.[74]

Lastly, research has also found that the amount of angiotensin II and aldosterone hormones can be double or triple in obese patients when compared to that of non-obese individuals.[74] As previously discussed, these are two hormones triggered by the body during times of stress to increase blood pressure. Obesity causes an abnormal amount of these hormones, which keeps blood pressure elevated.

Diet and Lifestyle

Studies have found that continued sedentary behavior, such as driving, watching television, and sitting behind the computer for extended periods, can lead to a higher risk of developing hypertension.[85] To combat this, frequent exercise is recommended. Exercise has two effects on blood pressure. Immediately following exercise, blood pressure is lowered for about 24 hours. While sustained effects can lessen blood pressure for days, months, or even years so long as you exercise frequently.[86] Studies found individuals who maintained a regular exercise routine lowered their risk of hypertension by 26 to 28 percent.[86]

A high sodium diet is also a risk factor for primary hypertension. Unfortunately, there is no way to predict sodium sensitivity.[18] While the general functions of kidneys are the same in all of us, there are slight differences that vary from person to person. One such variation is sodium sensitivity. Those who are salt-sensitive will find that even a small amount of sodium can wreak havoc with their blood pressure.[74] As we saw from the DASH trials, blood pressure decreased with an increase in fruits and vegetables but was lowered even more when paired with a reduced sodium intake.

Research has shown that excessive alcohol intake, better known as repeated binge drinking, can lead to alcohol-induced hypertension. This happens due to alcohol's effect on angiotensin II, which then increases blood pressure.[87] But how much is too much? The National Institute on Alcohol Abuse and Alcoholism (NIAAA) defines binge drinking as typically four or more drinks within two hours for women and five or more drinks within two hours for men. Drinking heavily and regularly can also cause strokes, irregular heartbeats, and heart attack.[18]

Smoking can cause many preventable diseases and conditions. But did you know that smoking affects your blood pressure? According to the American Heart Association, smoking has not been directly linked as a cause of high blood pressure.[88] But research has shown that each smoking session spikes blood pressure for a few minutes afterward. The nicotine in cigarettes increases blood pressure by triggering the sympathetic nervous system. Smoking also contributes to the stiffening of the arteries and body inflammation, which are both contributors to cardiovascular disease.[54]

While dehydration is not a risk factor for hypertension, staying hydrated is highly recommended. Your body will raise blood pressure as a response to dehydration. So, ensuring you stay hydrated maintains blood volume, which directly benefits your heart and blood pressure.[89] The amount of water you need varies daily based on your activities. The more you perspire, the more you need to replenish the fluids you lost. You can gauge your level of hydration based on the color of your urine. The darker the color, the more dehydrated you are.[89]

Demographics

If you have family members with hypertension, there is a possibility that it can run in the family. Researchers have learned a lot about hypertension through genetic research and found that there are specific genes responsible for increased blood pressure that are transferred from parents to their children.[90] Studies also suggest that specific changes in DNA structure in a fetus can make them susceptible to hypertension when they grow older.[91] The third form of hypertension through genetics is called monogenic hypertension. It occurs as a result of a genetic mutation of a single gene that triggers the kidneys to reabsorb a large amount of salt and water, increasing blood pressure.[74] This is very rare and affects only 1% of the hypertensive population.

Your ethnicity may also indicate how likely you are to get hypertension. A more significant percentage of African Americans have hypertension compared to the Asian, Hispanic, and Caucasian populations.[91] African Americans not only have higher blood pressure on average but also tend to get it at a young age.[91] Another factor is gender. At an older age, men are diagnosed with hypertension much earlier than women, as early as forty-five years of age. Where women tend to develop high blood pressure as much as seven or ten years later.[18] But, once women reach the age of sixty-five, there are more women than men with hypertension.[18]

Speaking of age. As you get older, you are prone to become more salt-sensitive.[74] There is also a recent increase in children and teens with hypertension caused by early-age obesity.[18] If you became hypertensive in your later years, around the ages of 50 to 60 years old, your high blood pressure is most likely caused by the natural stiffening and thickening of your blood vessels.[91] Recent statistics reported 65 percent of people develop hypertension over the age of sixty. This means by the age of 55, if you do not have high blood pressure yet, there is still a 90 percent chance of developing hypertension.[18]

Health Risks from Hypertension

Having hypertension means your blood is continuously pumping at a high pressure for an extended time. If it remains unmanaged for years, the extra pressure can wear out your blood vessels leading to permanent damage to the vessels in your heart, eyes, brain, and kidneys.[18] High blood pressure also stretches your blood vessels, which can cause ruptures, scar tissue, and tears. These lead to a buildup of blood cells, cholesterol, and plaque, which in turn leaves less room for blood flow. Al of this causes blood pressure to increase even more.[18]

As a secondary consequence, plaque can travel to other parts of your blood vessels and block blood flow to essential organs such as your eyes, heart, brain, and kidneys. This is why hypertension can lead to aneurysms, eye damage, paralysis, stroke, chronic kidney disease, vascular dementia, peripheral artery disease, and heart attacks.[92] Hypertension is known as a "silent killer" since many people go undiagnosed because there are no apparent symptoms when they start developing high blood pressure. For these individuals who are unaware, they usually don't find out about their condition until a heart attack or stroke occurs years later.

One in three Americans, which is about 75 million people, have hypertension and many do not know it. Only one in four of those with hypertension have it under control.[93] Reading about the consequences of uncontrolled hypertension is scary, but use this information as motivation to change your life and take control of your blood pressure. If you have read this book up to this point, take comfort in the fact that you are already well on your way say goodbye to high blood pressure!

CHAPTER ELEVEN

Shopping for DASH

From here on out, we suggest making a habit of turning food products around to read the nutrition label whenever you are grocery shopping. Not everything will have a nutrition label of course, such as fresh fruits and vegetables. But you should find nutrition labels on most preprepared meals, dried goods, canned food, packaged snacks, and drinks. You can use the nutrition label to make informed purchase decisions and to help you find products to fit your DASH needs. On the next page is a sample nutrition label of a generic can of black beans. We will use this example as we discuss the different parts of a nutrition label, and what to look for when finding DASH-friendly products.

Servings

The serving size indicates either the recommended amount to eat or the typical amount someone would eat in one sitting. The servings per container are the total number of serving sizes in the container. In the example label for the black beans, one serving size is 1/2 cup, but there are 3.5 servings in the entire can. It is important not to skip this part of the label. The nutrition label reflects information for just one serving. If your portion size is larger than the listed serving size, you will need to do some math to get an accurate measurement of your nutrients.

Nutrition Facts	
3.5 servings per container **Serving Size**	**½ cup (125 g)**
Amounts Per Serving **Calories**	**110**
	% Daily Value
Total Fat 0g	**0%**
Saturated Fat 0g	**0%**
Trans Fat 0g	
Polyunsaturated 0g	
Monounsaturated 0g	
Cholesterol 0mg	**0%**
Sodium 130mg	**5%**
Total Carbohydrate 20g	**7%**
Dietary Fiber 6g	**24%**
Sugars 2g	
includes 0g Added Sugars	
Protein 7g	
Vitamin D 0mcg	**0%**
Calcium 40mg	**4%**
Iron 1mg	**6%**
Potassium 440mg	**10%**

If you decide to eat one cup of black beans, you would need to multiply all the numbers on the label by two. Therefore, there are 110 calories for a 1/2-cup serving, but there are 220 calories for a one-cup serving. If you want to eat the entire can of black beans, you would multiply all the numbers by 3.5 to account for all the servings in the can. Thus, the whole can of beans contains 385 calories.

The percentage daily value shows how much of your recommended daily nutrients are met by each serving. The recommended values are based on a general 2,000 calorie diet. In our opinion, these numbers are rather arbitrary but do provide a quick reference without analyzing the amounts of grams in each nutrient. We recommended rather taking the time to look at the grams per serving to inform your decision.

Calories

Calories are what we refer to when we talk about the energy or fuel our bodies use. All foods are broken down into energy and have a caloric value based on how much protein, carbs, and fat are in them. Our bodies need a certain number of calories to function daily. That's why we eat.

Taking a look at the calories can be helpful in your diet but is not the ultimate and only information to consider, especially for DASH. Even though we determined your daily caloric needs for weight loss in Chapter 5, it was only to find your ideal DASH plan. We do not count calories on the DASH diet and rather focus on lowering saturated fats, trans fats, sodium, and added sugar, and increasing fiber, heart-healthy fats, vitamins, and minerals.

Total Fat

The total fat section of the nutrition label shows the total amount of dietary fat in that serving size. This is then further broken down into the various types of dietary fat. Most of the time, you will see saturated and trans fats listed, but you will also find monounsaturated (MUFAs) and polyunsaturated (PUFAs) fats if the food contains them. While there are no MUFAs or PUFAs in black beans, you will see it on something like a bottle of avocado oil. One serving size of a tablespoon of avocado oil contains 1.5 grams of PUFAs and 10 grams of MUFAs.

While you are shopping with DASH recommendations in mind, look for products with little or no saturated and trans fats. Both fats can increase your LDL cholesterol, and trans fats can also raise your triglycerides.[94] [95] On the other hand, do opt for products with MUFAs and PUFAs. These unsaturated fats lower LDL cholesterol and increase good HDL cholesterol. They can also improve your insulin if you have insulin resistance.[96] [97]

Cholesterol

Dietary cholesterol has made the news quite a bit over the years and was believed to be a major role player in heart disease. But studies have found that dietary cholesterol has little effect on coronary heart disease risk, especially compared to saturated and trans fats.[98] It might still be of concern to individuals with diabetes. Observational studies suggest dietary cholesterol may increase the risk of heart disease for those with diabetes,[99] while experimental studies have shown the opposite to be true.[100] Due to the conflicting results, we suggest you err on the side of caution if you do happen to be diabetic.

Our bodies also naturally produce cholesterol, so it is not an essential nutrient we must include in our diets. In terms of food sources, cholesterol is only found in meat and animal-based products. Fruits, vegetables, grains, and other fresh produce are all naturally cholesterol-free.

Sodium

We've covered sodium in detail in Chapter 3. Packaged foods usually contain a fair amount of sodium to improve flavor and extend the shelf life of products. Sodium functions as a preservative, flavor enhancer, thickener, stabilizer, and acid controller.[101] When looking at sodium on the nutrition label, pay special attention to the serving size. A snack-sized bag of chips might state that it contains 390 mg of sodium. But if the serving size is half of the bag, the entire bag of chips contains a substantial 780 mg of sodium. As you can see, the serving size makes a significant difference if you are trying to manage your sodium intake.

You should be tracking your sodium intake to ensure you stay below 2,300 mg or 1,500 mg per day, depending on the severity of your blood pressure. But, measuring sodium goes beyond the amount of table salt you add to your meals. Sodium can be found in packaged food, baked goods, pre-seasoned meat, canned vegetables, condiments, cheese, bottled sauces, salad dressings, cured meat, pickled produce, chips, frozen dinners, sports drinks, soups, broths, and more. Since sodium is both a preservative and flavor enhancer, it is no surprise you will find it in many packaged and processed foods. Let's look at ways you can identify sodium on packaging labels.

Nutrition labels list ingredients in descending order according to their weight. If you spot salt in the first few listed ingredients, chances are the product may contain a lot of sodium. Sodium comes in many forms. Of course, anything with the word sodium is a giveaway, such as sodium caseinate, sodium citrate, and sodium propionate.[18] Sodium is also found in baking powder, baking soda, soy sauce, teriyaki sauce, and monosodium glutamate (MSG).[18] If you purchase brined meat, it will also contain sodium since brining is the process of submerging the meat in salt and water.

As food companies are slowly decreasing the amount of sodium in their products, their labels will generally reflect this change. Seeing food labels with "low-sodium" or "reduced sodium" is common, but what do all these terms mean for someone with hypertension? The wording "unsalted" or "no salt added" means there was no salt added when the food was processed. When a product is labeled "salt-free" or "sodium-free" there are no more than 5 mg of sodium in each serving. However, some food can still contain naturally occurring sodium. Products labeled "very low sodium" have less than 35 mg per serving, and "low sodium" contains less than 140 mg per serving.[102]

The next category of sodium wording compares original products to sodium-altered counterparts. You will find this in foods such as broths, soups, canned beans, nuts, and other snacks. When a label says "reduced sodium" or "less sodium", it contains about 25% less sodium than the original version. Going one step further, "lightly salted" contains about 50% less sodium in comparison.[102] The original may contain a great deal of sodium, so the lightly salted versions can still be inappropriate for a low-sodium diet. Therefore, reading the nutrition labels for the altered products is very important.

Total Carbohydrates

Carbohydrates are the only macronutrient that is not essential in a diet. Our bodies are capable of producing the energy it needs from protein and fat in the absence of carbs. Despite this, carbs are still regarded as the primary source of glucose, energy, and fiber for our bodies. On the nutrition label, you will find two types of carbohydrates listed: dietary fiber and sugar.

Fiber can be divided into soluble and insoluble fiber. Soluble fiber dissolves in water and slows the digestion of foods. Insoluble fiber does not dissolve and assists in getting foods through the digestive system. As you shop at the grocery store, opt for food with fiber as much as possible. You will find this in food products containing whole grains, fruits, vegetables, whole wheat, beans, nuts, and seeds. The current recommendation for fiber is 25g per day for women and 31g per day for men.[103] So why is fiber important for DASH and weight loss? A diet rich in fiber prevents heart disease and obesity, and it helps you feel fuller for longer, which can assist in weight loss.

When looking at sugar, you will of course want to find foods that are low in sugar. But some foods have sugars naturally, like fruit and milk-based products. To cater to this, new nutrition labels have now added an "Added Sugars" category to distinguish between naturally occurring sugars and added sugar. Take yogurt as an example. Yogurt contains a natural sugar called lactose, which will be counted as "Sugars". Many brands add sugary ingredients to sweeten yogurt even more. On older nutrition labels, this will be counted as "Sugars" as well. But on newer labels, it will have its own "Added Sugars" category.

Be sure to always check the ingredient list if you are unsure whether a product contains added sugars. These sugars can appear as brown sugar, cane sugar, corn sweetener, corn syrup, dextrose, fructose, glucose, high-fructose corn syrup, honey, lactose, malt syrup, maple syrup, maltose, molasses, raw sugar, sucrose, and white sugar.[103] Even though lactose and fructose are naturally occurring sugars in milk products and fruit, respectively, they can still be used as an additive, in which case they will be listed in the ingredient list.

Protein

Protein is an important nutrient when it comes to fitness and exercise. It is an essential macronutrient and comprises of smaller molecules known as amino acids. Essential amino acids cannot be synthesized or created by our bodies and have to be taken in with our diets by consuming protein sources. Non-essential amino acids are equally as important, but our bodies can create them on their own. Protein is critical in keeping our skin, bones, organs, and muscles functioning, as well as building and retaining muscle.

There are many sources of protein (dairy, meat, legumes, etc.), but are some better than others? The answer is yes and no. There is no difference in the quality of protein when consuming mixed proteins at the general levels we would consume them. The source of protein would only make a difference in the case of a single source consumed in very low quantities. Think of impoverished countries where food is scarce. All high protein sources are more than sufficient in meeting the amino acid requirements of adults.[104] So, when it comes to protein, the source of protein doesn't really matter. But the choice of protein does matter when considering the other nutrients such as vitamins, minerals, fat, and carbohydrates.[104]

Following the DASH diet will ensure you eat an adequate amount of protein since you will be focusing on lean protein sources. Nutrition labels for products like packaged meat, fish, milk, and nuts will also be high in protein. As we have mentioned previously, if you are on a plant-based diet, ensure you look for higher protein content in your foods, to ensure you get an adequate amount of protein.

Vitamins and Minerals

Food with vitamin D, calcium, iron, and potassium are nutritional bonuses! Calcium and potassium are both heart-healthy minerals and great for lowering blood pressure, which we discussed in Chapter 3.

As you know by now, the DASH diet is rich in fiber, heart-healthy fats, vitamins, and minerals. It also keeps saturated fats, trans fats, added sugar, and sodium to a minimum. You can quickly identify these items on a nutrition label by following our guidelines above. Being able to determine which foods are DASH-friendly based on their nutrition labels will set you on the path to DASH success. Use every grocery trip as an opportunity to practice reading nutrition labels, and it will become second nature in no time.

CHAPTER TWELVE

Flex Your Culinary Muscles

If you are a kitchen novice looking to pick up a few new skills to make the DASH diet a success in your life, this section is for you! Working your way to becoming a kitchen warrior will be a freeing experience as you gain control over the food and nutrition you put in your body. It will take some dedication to put in the time and effort to learn and grow, but it will be worth it. Remember, if a cooking session didn't go well, just try again! Over time, you will be able to tweak recipes to your taste and learn new flavors along the way. Cooking can be a lot of fun and a rewarding experience.

In this chapter, we will review essential cooking tools and food safety to help you feel comfortable when cooking. We will also look into meal planning, preparing food in advance, and essential tips for stocking your pantry, fridge, and freezer.

Essential Cooking Tools

Cooking doesn't require fancy tools. Although, you can get more elaborate as you advance your cooking skills or you have a sudden interest in acquiring fun kitchen gadgets. The following are essential items for a beginner's cook kit: a chef's knife, two cutting boards, a large skillet, one medium saucepan, a rectangular baking pan, a pot, a steamer, a colander, a set of measuring cups and spoons, a liquid measuring cup, a food thermometer, storage containers, and cooking utensils such as a wooden spoon, spatula, and tongs. These few items are an excellent foundation for cooking almost anything. Let's look at why.

A chef's knife is a standard knife that can cut through most meats and produce, so long as you keep it sharp by using a honing stick or a knife sharpener. Other knives are fun to have but not necessary. For cutting boards, we recommend having two. But also try getting them in different colors. Dedicate one board for cutting raw meats and the other for fresh and cooked ingredients. The two-board method ensures you will not accidentally cross-contaminate your produce or ready-to-eat foods with raw meats that contain bacteria.

Having a skillet, saucepan, pot, steamer, and baking pan gives you the freedom to fry, bake, make soup and grains, boil pasta, and steam fish and vegetables. A colander is a useful tool when you need to drain pasta or if you need to wash vegetables while prepping. Your choice of cooking utensils is a personal preference. A wooden spoon is great for stirring, a spatula helps you flip fish and eggs, and tongs give you the ease of grabbing and tossing ingredients. Having a set of measuring cups and spoons is needed when you follow recipes, but also have a liquid measuring cup. Measure dry ingredients with measuring cups and spoons, and measure wet ingredients, such as broth and water, with a liquid measuring cup to help with accuracy.

After cooking, you will need storage containers to put away the delicious food you made. They will be especially useful when you start meal prepping or batch cooking. When shopping for storage containers, try to find ones that are safe for both refrigeration and freezing. Plastic containers are affordable and come in larger quantities, but there is a downside though. They stain and hang onto odor. Glass containers, on the other hand, do not stain or retain odors, but they are more expensive and can break easier than plastic.

Once cooking becomes an integral part of your life, you can invest in an intermediate home cook's toolkit. Extras such as a salad spinner, grill pan, food processor, and blender will open a new repertoire of recipes and cooking possibilities!

Food Safety

Understanding the basics of food safety and sanitation allows you to cook confidently, knowing you are keeping yourself and others you cook for safe. Food poisoning and surprise appearances of hair and debris in the final product are all preventable! You can find bacteria in many types of food, and one of them is meat. They grow at exponential rates at room temperature, therefore storing raw meat in the fridge or freezer is a necessity because it slows bacterial growth, and cooking the meat to high enough temperatures will kill off the bacteria.[105]

Different types of bacteria live on different types of meat, which is why the proper temperatures differ amongst poultry, beef, pork, and fish. Whenever you cook meat, use a food thermometer to make sure it has reached the appropriate internal temperature. Serving undercooked meat can cause food poisoning. To check the temperature, stick the thermometer into the thickest part of the flesh. All poultry, like turkey and chicken, need to reach a temperature of 165 F. Beef, pork, lamb, veal, ham, fish, and shellfish are safe at 145 F. Ground poultry needs to reach 165 degrees F and in contrast, all other types of ground meats need to hit 160 F.[106]

We can cause many different foodborne illnesses by not practicing proper handwashing, coughing or sneezing into food, handling food while sick, and cross-contamination.[105] Wash your hands with soap and warm water thoroughly before you cook and after handling raw meat. If you need to cough or sneeze, cover it with your arm and away from the food. We covered cross-contamination already. The solution is to have two cutting boards: one for raw meat and one for cooked food and fresh fruit and vegetables.

As for contaminants in food, you can tuck your hair away in a chef's hat or baseball cap to keep hair out of the food. It is also ideal for nails to be trimmed and clean with no nail polish, so debris and nail polish bits do not find their way onto the plate. Once the prepared food is ready, allow the food to cool down, then store it in the fridge or freezer within two hours of cooking.[105] Since bacteria reproduce at room temperature, ensuring food is stored soon after cooking will keep it safe. Practicing food safety and sanitation is an essential skill as a home cook. We don't want your excellent effort to go wasted if the food becomes unsafe to eat.

Stocking the Pantry, Fridge, and Freezer

Keeping your pantry, fridge, and freezer stocked with staple ingredients is terrific for having food on hand at all times. Stock your pantry with your favorite whole grains, nuts, seeds, beans, dried fruit, canned produce and salmon, and pouches of tuna. These items are exceptional since they have a long shelf-life. Do shop for items that are unsalted, very low-sodium, and have no added sugar. A pantry is also an opportunity to store your pick of herbs, spices, seasonings, and cooking oils. In a dry, cool area of your pantry or cabinet, store potatoes, garlic, and onions.

A freezer allows you to stock up on frozen fruits, vegetables, fish, meat, and grains that you can reheat or use in a recipe or a smoothie. Buying frozen produce at the grocery store is a fantastic option since they are frozen soon after picking and retain a lot of their nutrients. Some fresh fruits and vegetables lose their nutrition over time when they travel long distances and spend time sitting in the grocery store display. Frozen items also keep a few months longer than refrigerated food, so it is beneficial to have your freezer stocked with your favorite DASH items.

It takes more effort to maintain perishable items and a refrigerator can require restocking almost weekly. Keep your milk, eggs, yogurt, vegetables, fruit, salad dressings, meats, fish, leftovers, and prepped meals in the fridge. It helps keep your food lasting longer by a few days to a week. It might be helpful to put a label on each item to note the day it expires or note the day it was cooked. This way you can ensure you eat them before they spoil. If you have some food you know you will not be able to eat within a few days, go ahead and freeze them for a later time.

Meal Planning

Making an effort to plan your meals and snacks ahead of time is a great way to keep you on track with the DASH diet. Think about ways you will season your food with minimal salt. Instead of salt and pepper-crusted chicken or salmon, try lemon pepper chicken or orange rosemary salmon. Make your grains exciting with a squeeze of lime and chopped cilantro. Flavor your veggies with aromatic garlic and onions, and a sprig of thyme. The flavor possibilities are endless, so put on your exploration hat and try new combinations.

As for adding more fruits and vegetables to your meals, you don't always need to make them a side or a salad. You can throw them into your main course. Such as adding spinach, cabbage, or broccoli to soups, some kale in a smoothie, bell peppers and zucchini in pasta, and using strawberries or mandarin oranges as salad toppers. On occasion, you may be in the mood to try something new. Scope out a fruit or vegetable or a different type of fish you have never tried before. Then bring it home and try it in a simple recipe. Developing your palate keeps it exciting in the kitchen, and helps you grow your list of favorite DASH-friendly ingredients.

When shopping, you can maximize your groceries and reduce food waste by planning meals that use similar ingredients. For example, you can use half an onion for chili and the other half for a stir-fry, or use a package of chicken breasts for both tacos and soup. Before you go shopping, see what ingredients you have at home already and make a grocery list of the remaining items you need. Plan for leftovers, as well! If you are feeding additional family members, make sure you double or triple recipes as required.

Meal Prepping

Meal prepping may feel like a pain, but it is one of the best ways to set yourself up for success. If you live a busy life, finding the willpower to cook a fresh meal every day may not be a realistic scenario. Finding the discipline to dedicate time for food prepping will make the week ahead of you much more comfortable. You will have healthy, prepared meals and snacks in the fridge, which means less time thinking about food and more time doing other things that matter in your life.

One way to meal prep is to prepare a couple of whole meals in advance and refrigerate them for reheating at mealtime. When preparing meals, choose a couple of recipes you would like to eat during the week and that you are familiar with. Choose recipes that make use of different cooking methods so you don't have three or four meals needing the oven at the same time. Usually, one oven meal and two stovetop meals work well together.

When preparing meals, start with the recipes that require the longest cook times first. Another timesaver tip is to check your recipes for shared ingredients and prepare them at the same time. Such as chopping onions and tomatoes for a stew and a salad. Once the meals are made, store them in BPA-free microwaveable containers in the fridge for safe storage and easy reheating. Be mindful to refrigerate the meals within two hours after cooking, and consume them within three to four days.[107]

Another way to meal prep is preparing ingredients in advance. The idea is to cook a large number of ingredients and freeze it for later use. Or you can put it away in the fridge to eat throughout the week. For example, if you know you will not be motivated every day to prep and cook veggies, make a large batch of roasted vegetables or sauteed greens. Store them away and eat them as a side for the majority of your meals. You can apply this to many foods and ingredients you know you will need or want to eat during the week, such as rice, grains, fruit salad, pasta, and chicken breasts.

Let's say you're in the mood for ground beef. You can cook a batch of ground beef and store it in the fridge to add to tacos, pasta, or chili as you please. Batch cooking ingredients is a great way to save time and mix and match your protein, grains, and veggies so your meals can stay interesting throughout the week. If you set aside time to prep meals or ingredients in advance, you will have enough food for each meal time and will not have to worry about spending hours preparing meals after a long, tiring workday.

CHAPTER THIRTEEN

Final Thoughts

Implementing the DASH diet into your life will take time. Don't let the information from this guide overwhelm you. It will be here for you whenever you need it. You already took the hardest step, which was to recognize that you needed to make a change in your life to manage your hypertension. Take time to understand the breakdown of the DASH diet. Then practice building DASH-friendly meals, take every opportunity at the grocery store to read nutrition labels, and track your sodium. Develop your cooking skills, get more active, destress when you can, and remember to use the resources available to prepare yourself whenever you go out to eat. The more you practice and try, the easier it will be!

As you prepare for the DASH diet and other lifestyle changes, find joy in the little things. Find excitement in trying a new DASH recipe, or a new type of exercise. Be proud of every step you take, from managing your sodium intake to preparing each DASH-friendly meal. The ability to control your blood pressure and your weight lies in your hands. Believe in yourself and your hard work will pay off!

Maintaining Your Blood Pressure

Once you reach a healthy blood pressure, you must maintain the DASH diet and other lifestyle changes to prevent your blood pressure from increasing again. Once you have hypertension, you have it for life. Luckily, maintaining the DASH diet and regular physical activity will help you manage your blood pressure. Since the DASH diet will eventually be a permanent lifestyle change, take what you learn from this book and implement changes slowly. Start tracking your sodium intake, adding a few fruits and vegetables to some meals, and move your body a little bit. As you get used to that, you can start adding more changes until diet and physical activity becomes second nature.

The key to success with the DASH diet is becoming a home cook. Handpicking your ingredients, making purchase decisions based on the information on nutrition labels, and prepping and cooking your meals put the ultimate control in your hands. Since fast food and restaurant food tend to be high in sodium, added sugar, and saturated fats, it is best to reduce the number of times you eat out. On the occasions that you do dine out, practice mindful eating techniques, and follow the tips we provided.

Remember to continue routine checkups and to share your progress with your doctor. Continue antihypertensive medications as prescribed, but keep the conversation open about potentially reducing or eliminating them as your blood pressure and health improve. Also, consider working with a Registered Dietitian who can help you set up goals and provide any nutrition-related support and education you may desire. Keeping your health professionals up-to-date on your progress is essential in managing the condition and preventing potential health risks caused by hypertension, such as kidney disease, heart attacks, and eye damage.

You may fall off the bandwagon at times but never let it deter you from climbing back on. Life, understandably, has many obstacles, but know that you can always return to the DASH diet. You can start back up as soon as the next meal or the following day. If you start feeling discouraged or need motivation while you are making these lifestyle changes, remember why you wanted to stop hypertension. Also consider involving your friends, family, or co-workers in your journey. A support network and accountability buddy can help you reach your goals and maintain them.

Maintaining Your Weight

Once you reach the right weight for yourself and your health, it will be time to look at maintenance. Successful weight maintenance is defined as gaining less than 6.6 pounds, and less than 1.6 inches on your waist, in two years.[55] Maintaining your weight may be the hardest factor in the weight-loss equation. But if you've been keeping up with the DASH diet and the recommendations in this book, maintaining your physique will not require any more effort on your part. The good news is that you will be able to increase your daily servings somewhat, now that you don't need to be in a calorie deficit.

If you recall, we had specific tables in Chapter 5 that guided you on how many daily calories you need to lose weight. We've adjusted those tables to now reflect the ideal number of calories needed to maintain your weight once you feel you've reached the ideal number on the scale. The tables on the following pages work in the same way as the ones you used before, simply choose the table for women or men, then your age range, current weight, and current activity level. We will then use this calorie number to choose a new DASH plan.

Now that you have your new number of daily calories, we'll choose a matching DASH diet plan. The DASH plans in the table on the following pages are the same as the ones you are familiar with. Simply choose the closest matching calorie group based on your new calorie number. Remember, if your recommended calories span across two groups, choose the lower group if your weight falls on the lower end of the weight range in the previous table, and choose the higher group if you're on the higher end of the weight range. Refer to Chapter 5 for a detailed example.

Your new plan will prescribe exactly how many servings of each food group you need per day to maintain your current weight. However, each person's physique and daily calorie needs are unique, and simply jumping to the new meal plan might not work for everyone. For the best results, we suggest slowly increasing your number of servings from your current weight loss meal plan to the new maintenance meal plan over the course of a few months.

Pay special attention to your weight and waistline during this period when going from your current weight loss meal plan to the new maintenance meal plan. If you feel you are gaining any weight or inches around your waist before reaching your maintenance servings, reduce the servings slightly and stay on this level. This will then be your personal maintenance meal plan going forward. Maintaining a certain level of physical activity will also aid in maintaining the weight you lost. Losing weight is hard, and you most certainly do not want to do it again!

Daily calorie requirements for maintenance (women)

Age	Weight (lbs.)	Sedentary	Lightly Active	Moderately Active	Very Active
19 – 29	up to 119	1400	1500	1700	1800
	120-139	1400 – 1500	1500 – 1600	1700 – 1800	1800 – 2000
	140-159	1500 – 1600	1600 – 1700	1800 – 2000	2000 – 2100
	160-199	1600 – 1800	1700 – 2000	2000 – 2200	2100 – 2400
	200+	1800	2000	2200	2400
30 – 39	up to 119	1300	1500	1600	1800
	120-139	1300 – 1400	1500 – 1600	1600 – 1800	1800 – 1900
	140-159	1400 – 1500	1600 – 1700	1800 – 1900	1900 – 2000
	160-199	1500 – 1700	1700 – 1900	1900 – 2100	2000 – 2300
	200+	1700	1900	2100	2300

Daily calorie requirements for maintenance (women)

Age	Weight (lbs.)	Sedentary	Lightly Active	Moderately Active	Very Active
40 – 49	up to 119	1300	1400	1600	1700
	120-139	1300 – 1400	1400 – 1500	1600 – 1700	1700 – 1800
	140-159	1400 – 1500	1500 – 1600	1700 – 1800	1800 – 1900
	160-199	1500 – 1700	1600 – 1800	1800 – 2100	1900 – 2200
	200+	1700	1800	2100	2200
50+	up to 119	1200	1400	1500	1600
	120-139	1200 – 1300	1400 – 1500	1500 – 1700	1600 – 1800
	140-159	1300 – 1400	1500 – 1600	1700 – 1800	1800 – 1900
	160-199	1400 – 1600	1600 – 1800	1800 – 2000	1900 – 2200
	200+	1600	1800	2000	2200x

Daily calorie requirements for maintenance (men)

Age	Weight (lbs.)	Sedentary	Lightly Active	Moderately Active	Very Active
19 - 29	up to 149	1800	2000	2200	2400
	150 - 169	1800 - 1900	2000 - 2100	2200 - 2400	2400 - 2500
	170 - 199	1900 - 2100	2100 - 2300	2400 - 2500	2500 - 2700
	200 - 229	2100 - 2200	2300 - 2400	2500 - 2700	2700 - 2900
	230+	2200	2400	2700	2900
30 - 39	up to 149	1800	1900	2200	2300
	150 - 169	1800 - 1900	1900 - 2000	2200 - 2300	2300 - 2500
	170 - 199	1900 - 2000	2000 - 2200	2300 - 2500	2500 - 2700
	200 - 229	2000 - 2200	2200 - 2400	2500 - 2700	2700 - 2900
	230+	2200	2400	2700	2900

Daily calorie requirements for maintenance (men)

Age	Weight (lbs.)	Sedentary	Lightly Active	Moderately Active	Very Active
40 – 49	up to 149	1700	1900	2100	2300
	150 – 169	1700 – 1800	1900 – 2000	2100 – 2200	2300 – 2400
	170 – 199	1800 – 2000	2000 – 2100	2200 – 2400	2400 – 2500
	200 – 229	2000 – 2100	2100 – 2300	2400 – 2600	2600 – 2800
	230+	2100	2300	2600	2800
50+	up to 149	1700	1800	2100	2200
	150 – 169	1700 – 1800	1800 – 1900	2100 – 2200	2200 – 2400
	170 – 199	1800 – 1900	1900 – 2100	2200 – 2400	2400 – 2500
	200 – 229	1900 – 2100	2100 – 2300	2400 – 2600	2500 – 2700
	230+	2100	2300	2600	2700

DASH plans (daily servings per food group)

Daily calories	1,200	1,400	1,600	1,800	2,000	2,200	2,400	2,600	2,800
Whole grains	4 – 5	5 – 6	6	6	6 – 8	8 – 9	9 – 10	10 – 11	11 – 12
Vegetables	3 – 4	3 – 4	3 – 4	4 – 5	4 – 5	4 – 5	5 – 6	5 – 6	5 – 6
Fruit	3 – 4	4	4	4 – 5	4 – 5	5	5 – 6	5 – 6	5 – 6
Dairy	2 – 3	2 – 3	2 – 3	2 – 3	2 – 3	3	3	3	3
Meat, poultry and fish	3 or less	4 or less	4 or less	6 or less	6 or less	6 or less	6 or less	6 or less	6 – 9
Fats and oils	1	1	2	2 – 3	2 – 3	2 – 3	3	3	3 – 4
Nuts, seeds, beans & peas	3 per week	3 per week	3-4 pr week	4 per week	4-5 pr week	5-6 pr week	5-6 pr week	7 per week	7 per week
Sweets and treats	3 or less per week								
Sodium	2,300 mg								

CHAPTER FOURTEEN

Simply Delicious Recipes

We have lovingly created 30 flavorful recipes for you to try on your DASH journey, covering everything from chocolate peanut butter smoothies and buffalo turkey burgers to Caribbean jerk shrimp and vegan coconut curry. All recipes include step-by-step instructions with nutritional info. They are easy to prepare and 100% DASH-approved!

Most recipes were created to serve a family of four. If you are cooking for less or more, adjust the recipes accordingly if you are experienced in the kitchen. If scaling recipes is not something you are comfortable with, we suggest simply storing the leftovers in the fridge or freezer (see Chapter 12) for an easy lunch or dinner later in the week. A US Standard to Metric chart is also included at the back of this book for those not in the United States.

Breakfast & Smoothies

page

Savory Oatmeal 132

Southwest Sweet Potato Hash 134

Veggie Tofu Scramble 136

Tropical Pina Colada Smoothie 138

Chocolate Peanut Butter Smoothie 139

Berries & Greens Smoothie 140

Seafood & Poultry Mains

Chili Lime Baked Tilapia 142

Caribbean Jerk Shrimp 144

Baked Mango Avocado Salsa Salmon 146

Shredded Barbecue Chicken Bowls 148

Chicken Fajita Casserole 150

Buffalo Turkey Burgers with Sweet Potato Fries 152

Herbed Chicken Breast with Spicy Peanut Sauce 154

Salads & Soups

Chipotle Chicken Salad with Ranch Dressing 157

Summer Berry Salad with Strawberry Vinaigrette 160

Power Greens Salad with Honey Mustard Dressing 162

Shredded Chicken Tortilla Soup 164

Veggie Loaded Chili 166

Blended Carrot Ginger Soup 168

Vegetarian & Vegan Mains

	page
Greek Grain Bowl with Tzatziki	170
Vegan Tofu Stir Fry Bowl	173
Chickpea Salad Lettuce Wraps	176
Pesto and Roasted Veggie Pasta	178
Honey & Garlic Tempeh	180
Vegan Lentil Ragu with Spaghetti Squash	182
Vegan Thai Coconut Curry	184

Beef & Pork Mains

Seared Sirloin with Chimichurri Sauce	186
Sirloin & Veggie Kebabs with Garlic Yogurt Dip	188
Honey Mustard Pork Tenderloin	190
Pork Chops with Sweet Cinnamon Apples	192

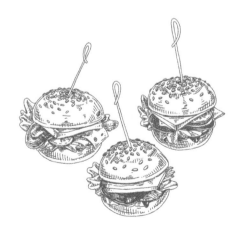

This savory oatmeal bowl will change the way you think about oatmeal! Nourishing, fiber-rich oats are accompanied by protein-rich egg whites, creamy avocado, and bright sauteed peppers. This traditionally sweet breakfast option just got a savory upgrade, and it's ready to keep you satisfied and fueled all morning long!

SAVORY OATMEAL

SERVINGS: 4 | PREP TIME: 5 min | COOK TIME: 10 min
SODIUM PER SERVING: 271 mg

1½ cups rolled oats

2 cups water

6 egg whites

1 medium, ripe avocado

½ cup cherry tomatoes

1 red bell pepper

⅓ large white onion, about ½ cup

1 tbsp olive oil

¼ tsp freshly ground black pepper

½ tsp onion salt

¼ tsp salt

1   Preheat a medium-sized skillet with oil to medium heat. Slice peppers and onions into strips about 1/4 inch thick. Add to pan, stirring occasionally. Cook until tender, about 4-5 minutes.

2   In a medium-sized pot, combine oats, water, onion salt, and egg whites. Bring to a boil then reduce to low heat, in order to simmer. Cook, stirring frequently, about 3-4 minutes or until thick and creamy.

3 Peel and slice avocado and halve the tomatoes. Portion oats into four bowls, top with pepper and onion mixture, avocado slices, tomatoes, salt and pepper, and enjoy.

Nutrition Facts per Serving

Servings 4 | Calories 244 | Total Fat 12 g | Saturated Fat 2 g
Monounsaturated Fat 6 g | Polyunsaturated Fat 1 g | Trans Fat 0 g
Cholesterol 0 mg | Sodium 271 mg | Total Carbohydrate 21 g
Dietary Fiber 7 g | Sugars 3 g | Protein 11 g

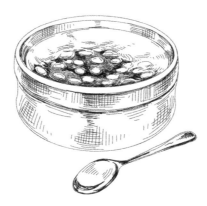

This southwest sweet potato hash is loaded. Sweet and crispy sweet potatoes, protein-packed ground chicken and eggs, spinach for a micronutrient boost, and warm and flavorful spices make this dish both nourishing and layered with flavor.

SOUTHWEST SWEET POTATO HASH

SERVINGS: 4 | PREP TIME: 5 min | COOK TIME: 20 min
SODIUM PER SERVING: 181 mg

1 medium sweet potato

½ pound lean ground chicken

⅓ cup white onion

2 cup spinach

2 eggs

½ tsp onion salt

1 tbsp cumin

1 tbsp chili powder

1 tbsp olive oil

1 Caramelize onions. Preheat a well-seasoned cast-iron skillet to medium-low heat with olive oil. Slice the onions into thin wedges and separate the layers to create thin strips. Add to the pan, stirring every couple of minutes, allow onions to slowly begin to caramelize and become brown in color, about 12 minutes. If the onions stick at any point, add a tablespoon of water. They will continue to caramelize throughout the entire cooking process.

2 Cook chicken. Increase the heat to medium. Add ground chicken, onion salt, cumin, and chili powder to the pan, stirring to break up the meat. Let the chicken brown completely, about 6 minutes.

3 Prepare the sweet potatoes by slicing them into 1/2 inch cubes. Add the cubed potatoes to the skillet and mix with the ground meat. Add about 1/3 cup of water, cover, and allow to cook until tender, about 10 minutes. Stir occasionally to achieve browning on all sides of your sweet potatoes.

4 In a small bowl, whisk together the eggs. Create a well in the skillet by moving the sweet potatoes to the sides, and adding the eggs. Stir frequently in the well until cooked through, about 3-4 minutes. Mix with the remaining skillet.

5 Add spinach, stir until wilted, about 1-2 minutes. Serve!

Nutrition Facts per Serving

Servings 4 | Calories 198 | Total Fat 12 g | Saturated Fat 3 g
Monounsaturated Fat 3 g | Polyunsaturated Fat 0 g | Trans Fat 0 g
Cholesterol 135 mg | Sodium 181 mg | Total Carbohydrate 9 g
Dietary Fiber 2 g | Sugars 2 g | Protein 15 g

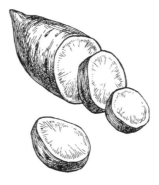

You won't believe this tofu scramble does not contain eggs! This vegetarian-friendly dish is loaded with plant-based protein, flavor, and colorful vegetables. Better yet, this recipe is easily customizable! Swap the vegetables for your seasonal favorites to mix it up.

VEGGIE TOFU SCRAMBLE

SERVINGS: 4 | PREP TIME: 5 min | COOK TIME: 10 min
SODIUM PER SERVING: 152 mg

19 oz firm tofu, strained

1 red bell pepper

¼ cup yellow onion

½ cup spinach

1 tbsp nutritional yeast

1 tsp turmeric powder

¼ tsp salt

Pinch black pepper

1 tbsp olive oil

1   Preheat a large skillet with olive oil to medium heat.

2   Finely dice the bell pepper and yellow onion, and add to the pan. Stirring frequently, sauté until they begin to soften and sweat, about 3-4 minutes.

3   Remove the tofu from the packaging and gently press with a kitchen towel to release excess moisture. Thoroughly pat dry. Note: use a cutting board that has ridges for collecting moisture to avoid a mess!

4   Add tofu, nutritional yeast, turmeric, salt, and pepper to the pan. Using a wooden spoon, break up the tofu and mix in the spices until the tofu reaches the consistency of scrambled eggs, and the spices are evenly distributed. Continue to cook until the tofu is heated through, about 2-3 minutes.

Note: if the tofu is not properly drained, cook an additional 2-3 minutes to evaporate excess water that may be released at this time.

5 Add spinach to the pan and stir frequently until it is wilted, about 1-2 minutes. Spoon onto four plates and serve!

Nutrition Facts per Serving

Servings 4 | Calories 104 | Total Fat 10 g | Saturated Fat 5 g

Monounsaturated Fat 2 g | Polyunsaturated Fat 0 g | Trans Fat 0 g

Cholesterol 0 mg | Sodium 152 mg | Total Carbohydrate 4 g

Dietary Fiber 2 g | Sugars 2 g | Protein 10 g

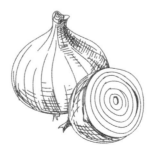

This smoothie is the tropical escape you need. Sweetened with frozen pineapple chunks and paired with protein-packed Greek yogurt, this combo is simple and delicious! Top it off with some unsweetened coconut flakes for some added texture and healthy fats.

TROPICAL PINA COLADA SMOOTHIE

SERVINGS: 4 | PREP TIME: 5 min | SODIUM PER SERVING: 30 mg

2 cups frozen pineapple chunks

1 cup plain Greek yogurt

1½ cup coconut milk, carton

½ cup unsweetened coconut flakes

1　Add pineapple, Greek yogurt, and coconut milk to a blender.

2　Blend until smooth, about 1 minute.

3　Portion into four glasses and top with coconut flakes. Enjoy!

Nutrition Facts per Serving

Servings 4 | Calories 157 | Total Fat 8 g | Saturated Fat 6 g
Monounsaturated Fat 0 g | Polyunsaturated Fat 0 g | Trans Fat 0 g
Cholesterol 8 mg | Sodium 30 mg | Total Carbohydrate 18 g
Dietary Fiber 3 g | Sugars 13 g | Protein 7 g

Chocolate and peanut butter is a classic combo that will never go out of style. Cocoa powder, peanut butter, and bananas are a dream team working together to create a smooth, creamy, and perfectly sweet breakfast that will nourish you in the morning, or even combat your sweet tooth during the day!

CHOCOLATE PEANUT BUTTER SMOOTHIE

SERVINGS: 4 | PREP TIME: 5 min | SODIUM PER SERVING: 71 mg

- 3 medium frozen bananas

- 3 tbsp cocoa powder

- 4 tbsp peanut butter, without salt

- 1 cup spinach

- 2 cups oat milk, unsweetened

1 Add all ingredients to a blender.

2 Blend until smooth, about 1 minute.

3 Portion into four glasses and enjoy!

Nutrition Facts per Serving

Servings 4 | Calories 201 | Total Fat 10 g | Saturated Fat 2 g
Monounsaturated Fat 0 g | Polyunsaturated Fat 0 g | Trans Fat 0 g
Cholesterol 0 mg | Sodium 71 mg | Total Carbohydrate 25 g
Dietary Fiber 5 g | Sugars 12 g | Protein 6 g

This berries and greens smoothie is full of micronutrients! Blueberries, strawberries, and kale create a beautifully nourishing breakfast that's lightly sweetened with honey, and boosted with plant-powered protein from hemp seeds.

BERRIES & GREENS SMOOTHIE

SERVINGS: 4 | PREP TIME: 5 min | SODIUM PER SERVING: 20 mg

1 cup frozen blueberries

1 cup frozen strawberries

¾ cup frozen kale

4 tbsp hemp seeds

1½ cup coconut milk

2 tbsp honey

1   Add all ingredients to a blender.

2   Blend until smooth, about 1 minute.

3   Portion into four glasses and enjoy!

Nutrition Facts per Serving

Servings 4 | Calories 158 | Total Fat 7 g | Saturated Fat 2 g
Monounsaturated Fat 1 g | Polyunsaturated Fat 4 g | Trans Fat 0 g
Cholesterol 0 mg | Sodium 20 mg | Total Carbohydrate 22 g
Dietary Fiber 3 g | Sugars 17 g | Protein 5 g

Which recipe is your favorite?

There is nothing that makes me happier than seeing readers use and enjoy my recipes. I have put a lot of time and love into crafting the recipes you see here, and I encourage you to try as many as you can to find which ones you enjoy the most. Consider showing off your culinary skills by sharing a photo of your favorite recipe on Amazon, it would absolutely warm my heart to see your creations!

This chili lime baked tilapia sits beautifully on tender bok choy and sweet caramelized onions. Each bite features a balanced spiced rub that's smokey, zesty, with just the right amount of heat. This delicious meal is ready in less than thirty minutes, making it perfect for a simple weeknight meal!

CHILI LIME BAKED TILAPIA

SERVINGS: 4 | PREP TIME: 10 min | COOK TIME: 15 min
SODIUM PER SERVING: 254 mg

4 tilapia filets

4 tbsp olive oil

1 tsp sea salt

4 tsp chili powder

2 tsp paprika

2 tsp garlic powder

4 tbsp lime juice

1 tsp lime zest

Additional lime wedges for garnish

4 heads baby bok choy

½ large sweet yellow onion

1   Preheat the oven to 350 Fahrenheit.

2   Create chili lime spice rub. Whisk together olive oil, salt, chili powder, paprika, garlic powder, lime juice, and lime zest to form a thick paste.

3   Pat tilapia dry before evenly spooning chili-lime paste onto each filet. Using your spoon or hands, spread the paste evenly over both sides of the filets.

4   Prepare the vegetables by slicing the bok choy into quarters lengthwise and slicing the yellow onion into wedges or rings.

5   Spread the vegetables in an even layer onto a foil-lined pan. Place the tilapia filet on top of the vegetable mixture to allow the chili lime paste to flavor the vegetables below throughout the cooking process. Bake for 15 minutes, or until tilapia is just flakey.

6   Serve hot and enjoy!

7   Optional: serve with lime wedges and squeeze over the dish just before enjoying!

Nutrition Facts per Serving

Servings 4 | Calories 303 | Total Fat 15 g | Saturated Fat 2 g
Monounsaturated Fat 10 g | Polyunsaturated Fat 2 g | Trans Fat 0 g
Cholesterol 50 mg | Sodium 254 mg | Total Carbohydrate 8 g
Dietary Fiber 3 g | Sugars 1 g | Protein 24 g

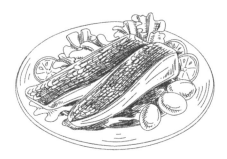

This Caribbean jerk shrimp with coconut rice and steamed peas brings tropical vibes to your home. A punchy spice rub brings some heat to each shrimp while coconut rice provides a creamy and lightly sweetened cool balance in every bite.

CARIBBEAN JERK SHRIMP

SERVINGS: 4 | PREP TIME: 10 min | COOK TIME: 25 min
SODIUM PER SERVING: 222 mg

Caribbean Jerk Shrimp

1 lb jumbo shrimp

2 tbsp olive oil

1 tsp smoked paprika

1 tsp brown sugar, packed

1 tsp oregano, dried

½ tsp garlic powder

½ tsp cayenne pepper

½ tsp cumin, ground

¼ tsp salt

¼ tsp black pepper, ground

pinch allspice, ground

Coconut Rice

1 cup white rice

15 oz can full-fat coconut milk

½ cup water

¼ cup coconut sugar

Steamed Peas

1 cup green peas

1 cup water

1   Prepare the rice by adding rice, coconut milk, water, and coconut sugar to a medium-sized pot and bring to a boil, stirring frequently. Once the mixture is boiling, cover and reduce heat to low. Allow to cook for 25 minutes, or until rice is tender and liquid is absorbed.

2   While the rice is cooking, prepare the shrimp. Combine the sugar, salt, herbs and spices, and half of the olive oil to form a rub. Pat the shrimp dry and toss with the spice mixture until evenly coated.

3   Preheat a saucepan to medium heat and lightly oil. Place the shrimp in the pan, taking care not to overcrowd the pan, so they can sear. Sear each side for 3-4 minutes, or until lightly charred. Remove from the heat and repeat until all of the shrimp is cooked.

4   Steam peas by placing them in a small pot with a lid and steamer basket. Fill the bottom of the steamer pot with water, cover, and cook on high for 4-5 minutes, or until the peas are bright in color and tender.

5   Assemble bowls by portioning rice, shrimp, and peas into four bowls and enjoy!

Nutrition Facts per Serving

Servings 4 | Calories 535 | Total Fat 27 g | Saturated Fat 17 g
Monounsaturated Fat 5 g | Polyunsaturated Fat 1 g | Trans Fat 0 g
Cholesterol 15 mg | Sodium 222 mg | Total Carbohydrate 55 g
Dietary Fiber 1 g | Sugars 16 g | Protein 15 g

Simple, fresh flavors create a bright and vibrant meal that is bursting with sweet citrus, savory salmon, sweet mango, and creamy avocado! Each component brings a new texture and flavor to the table, creating a party in your mouth with each bite. Let's dig in!

BAKED MANGO AVOCADO SALSA SALMON

SERVINGS: 4 | PREP TIME: 10 min | COOK TIME: 45 min
SODIUM PER SERVING: 230 mg

Salmon

16 oz salmon

1 tbsp olive oil

½ tsp kosher salt

¼ tsp black pepper

Cilantro Lime Rice

1 cup brown rice

1½ cup water

⅓ cup cilantro, packed

2 limes

Pinch of salt

Mango Avocado Salsa

1 red bell pepper

1 medium mango

1 medium avocado

¼ cup finely chopped red onion

½ lime, juice and zest

Optional: ½ jalapeno

1   Preheat the oven to 425 Fahrenheit.

2   Prepare the cilantro-lime rice by adding brown rice and water to a small pot. Bring to a boil, stir, cover, and reduce heat to low. Cook on low for 40-45 minutes, or until the water is absorbed.

3   While the rice is cooking, prepare the salmon. Add oil, salt, and pepper evenly to the filet. Place on a baking sheet lined with foil and bake for 15-18 minutes, or until the flesh is just flakey but not dried out. Note: you can use individual filets or one large filet for this recipe.

4   Prepare the mango avocado salsa. Remove the stem, seeds, and ribs from the bell pepper and optional jalapeno. Peel the mango and cut the flesh from the large pit in the center. Slice the avocado in half, remove the pit, and peel. Finely dice the peppers, meat of the mango, avocado, and red onion into pea-sized pieces. Combine in a large bowl and add the juice and zest of the lime, stir until combined.

5   When the rice is cooked, fluff with a fork. Roughly chop the cilantro, removing the stems, and juice the lime. Add cilantro, lime juice, and salt to the rice and stir to combine.

6   Assemble by portioning rice, salsa, and filets into four servings. Plate and enjoy while rice and salmon are hot.

Nutrition Facts per Serving

Servings 4 | Calories 417 | Total Fat 19 g | Saturated Fat 4 g
Monounsaturated Fat 6 g | Polyunsaturated Fat 1 g | Trans Fat 0 g
Cholesterol 57 mg | Sodium 230 mg | Total Carbohydrate 34 g
Dietary Fiber 5 g | Sugars 6 g | Protein 27 g

Enjoy this comforting dish with a warm and smoky barbecue sauce, crunchy baked carrots, chewy farro, and protein-packed chicken breast. This slow cooker chicken breast is juicy, tender, and flavorful. Enjoy every saucy bite!

SHREDDED BARBECUE CHICKEN BOWLS

SERVINGS: 4 | PREP TIME: 15 min | COOK TIME: 4 hours
SODIUM PER SERVING: 324 mg

Main Ingredients

16 oz chicken breast, about 4 small or 2 large

1 cup farro

3 cups water

6 large carrots

1 tbsp olive oil

¼ tsp kosher salt

Barbecue Sauce

½ yellow onion, finely diced

3 cloves garlic

6 oz can tomato paste, no salt added

5 tbsp balsamic vinegar

4 tbsp raw honey

1 tsp cumin

1 tbsp smoked paprika

½ tsp oregano

1   Prepare the barbecue sauce. Finely dice the yellow onion and mince the garlic. Combine onions, garlic, tomato paste, vinegar, honey, and spices to form a smooth sauce.

2   Add the chicken and barbecue sauce to a slow cooker and cook on high for about 3-4 hours, or until the chicken is cooked through and tender enough to shred with a fork. Optional: use a pressure cooker and cook on high for 25 minutes.

3   Shred chicken using two large forks and keep warm.

4   Once the chicken is cooked, preheat the oven to 425 Fahrenheit.

5   Prepare the carrot fries. Cut the carrots into thirds width-wise, then cut into quarters length-wise to form carrot strips. Lightly toss in oil and salt, then spread onto a baking sheet. Place carrot fries in the oven and bake for 15 minutes.

6   While the carrots are baking, prepare the farro. Bring water to a boil in a saucepan, add farro, reduce heat to low, cover and simmer for 10 minutes, then drain excess liquid.

7   Assemble into four bowls by creating a bed of farro, topping with carrot fries, and shredded chicken. Spoon additional barbecue sauce over the bowl to reach the desired saucy-ness. Enjoy warm!

Nutrition Facts per Serving

Servings 4 | Calories 469 | Total Fat 7 g | Saturated Fat 1 g
Monounsaturated Fat 3 g | Polyunsaturated Fat 1 g | Trans Fat 0 g
Cholesterol 65 mg | Sodium 508 mg | Total Carbohydrate 73 g
Dietary Fiber 7 g | Sugars 28 g | Protein 33 g

This chicken fajita casserole features sweet onions and bell peppers, warm aromatic spices, and protein-packed quinoa. Assemble this casserole with just a few simple steps, toss it in the oven, and enjoy a healthy and delicious dinner with minimal effort.

CHICKEN FAJITA CASSEROLE

SERVINGS: 4 | PREP TIME: 10 min | COOK TIME: 50 min
SODIUM PER SERVING: 467 mg

1 lb chicken breast

3 medium red bell peppers

½ large yellow onion

1 cup quinoa

1½ cups water

½ cup shredded cheddar cheese

1 tbsp chili powder

1½ tbsp cumin

1 tsp garlic powder

1 tsp onion powder

½ tsp salt

1   Preheat the oven to 350 Fahrenheit.

2   Prepare the vegetables by removing the stem, seeds, and ribs of the bell pepper. Slice the bell pepper and onion into long strips.

3   Slice the chicken into 1-inch cubes and toss in chili powder, cumin, garlic powder, onion powder, and salt until evenly coated.

4   In an 8x8 inch baking dish, add quinoa and water, add chicken in a single layer, and top with peppers and onions.

5 Cover with foil and bake for 45 minutes, or until chicken reaches 165 Fahrenheit.

6 Uncover, add cheese, and bake for an additional 10 minutes, or until cheese is melted and bubbly!

7 Portion casserole into four servings and enjoy warm!

Nutrition Facts per Serving

Servings 4 | Calories 268 | Total Fat 9 g | Saturated Fat 16 g

Monounsaturated Fat 5 g | Polyunsaturated Fat 6 g | Trans Fat 0 g

Cholesterol 81 mg | Sodium 467 mg | Total Carbohydrate 17 g

Dietary Fiber 2 g | Sugars 5 g | Protein 30 g

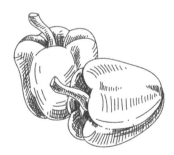

These juicy turkey burgers bring just the right amount of heat in every bite. Enjoy them on a whole wheat bun with thick tomato slices, cool cucumber, crisp romaine, and a side of sweet potato fries. Perfect for those days when you're not in the mood to cook and yearning for a good-ol' burger!

BUFFALO TURKEY BURGERS WITH SWEET POTATO FRIES

SERVINGS: 4 | PREP TIME: 15 min | COOK TIME: 25 min

SODIUM PER SERVING: 378 mg

Assembly Ingredients

1 beefsteak tomato

½ cup cucumber slices

4 large romaine leaves

4 whole-wheat buns

Turkey Burgers

1 lb ground turkey breast

¼ cup yellow onion, diced

1 tsp onion powder

⅓ cup parsley, packed

2 tbsp hot sauce, no sodium or low sodium

Sweet Potato Fries

2 medium-sized sweet potatoes

2 tbsp olive oil

Pinch of sea salt

1 Preheat the oven to 425 Fahrenheit.

2 Slice the sweet potatoes into 1/2 inch slices and toss in olive oil and sea salt. Spread into an even layer on a baking sheet and bake for 20-25 minutes, flipping halfway through.

3 While the sweet potatoes are baking, preheat a non-stick frying pan to medium-high heat and lightly grease with olive oil or cooking spray of choice.

4 Prepare the burgers by finely dicing the yellow onion and roughly chopping the parsley, removing stems. Combine the ground turkey, onions, parsley, salt, onion powder, and hot sauce until evenly combined. Form into four patties, and press to 1/2 inch thickness.

5 Place on a hot skillet and cook for 4-5 minutes per side, or until browned and cooked to an internal temperature of 165 Fahrenheit.

6 Slice the tomato and cucumber into thin disks.

7 Assemble the burgers by placing them in whole wheat buns and topping with tomato slices, cucumber slices, and lettuce. Enjoy with a side of sweet potato fries!

Nutrition Facts per Serving
Servings 4 | Calories 369 | Total Fat 10 g | Saturated Fat 1 g
Monounsaturated Fat 5 g | Polyunsaturated Fat 2 g | Trans Fat 0 g
Cholesterol 70 mg | Sodium 378 mg | Total Carbohydrate 39 g
Dietary Fiber 6 g | Sugars 7 g | Protein 37 g

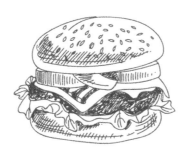

This herbed chicken breast with spicy peanut sauce is a bowl bursting with rich and diverse flavors. It is protein-packed and features smooth and creamy peanut sauce, whole grains, crisp cucumbers, and robust roasted broccoli. Enjoy this satiating and flavorful dish for lunch or dinner!

HERBED CHICKEN BREAST WITH SPICY PEANUT SAUCE

SERVINGS: 4 | PREP TIME: 30 min | COOK TIME: 35 min
SODIUM PER SERVING: 364 mg

Main Ingredients

1 cup quinoa

1 cup water

2 cups broccoli

1 tbsp olive oil

1 large cucumber, sliced

2 green onions, sliced

¼ cup unsalted peanuts

Herbed Chicken

1 lb chicken breast

2 tbsp brown sugar

2 tbsp olive oil

2 cloves garlic

1 tsp dried basil

1 tsp dried oregano

½ tsp sea salt

Peanut Sauce

¼ cup peanut butter, unsalted

¼ cup full fat coconut milk

2 tbsp low-sodium soy sauce

1 inch fresh ginger, minced

2 tsp brown sugar, packed

¼ to ½ tsp red pepper flakes

1 Prepare the chicken. Cut the chicken into 1-inch cubes and toss in olive oil, brown sugar, minced garlic, basil, oregano, and sea salt. Refrigerate to marinate for at least 30 minutes.

2 Preheat the oven to 425 Fahrenheit.

3 Chop the broccoli into small pieces, toss in olive oil, and spread onto a baking sheet. Roast in the oven for 15 min.

4 Prepare the quinoa. Combine the quinoa and water in a small pot and bring to a boil. Cover, reduce heat to low, and cook for 15 minutes, or until water is absorbed.

5 Preheat a large skillet to medium-high heat. Add the chicken to the pan and cook for 5-6 minutes per side, or until golden brown and cooked to an internal temperature of 165 Fahrenheit.

6 Prepare the peanut sauce by whisking together peanut butter, coconut milk, soy sauce, minced ginger, brown sugar, and red pepper flakes. Note: if the peanut butter is thick, microwave it for 15-20 seconds to soften before mixing. Additionally, add red pepper flakes to your preference!

7 Assemble bowls by portioning quinoa, broccoli, and chicken into four bowls. Top with sliced cucumbers, green onions, peanuts, and peanut sauce, and enjoy warm!

8 When shopping for soy sauce, look for low-sodium soy sauce that has about 300 mg or less of sodium per tablespoon. Alternatively opt for "coconut aminos" which has a similar flavor profile to soy sauce, albeit a little sweeter, but with much less sodium.

Nutrition Facts per Serving

Servings 4 | Calories 467 | Total Fat 27 g | Saturated Fat 18 g
Monounsaturated Fat 13 g | Polyunsaturated Fat 8 g | Trans Fat 0 g
Cholesterol 65 mg | Sodium 364 mg | Total Carbohydrate 27 g
Dietary Fiber 3 g | Sugars 10 g | Protein 32 g

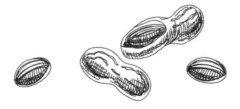

This chipotle chicken salad features protein-packed lean chicken breast with a powerful smokey spice rub that will have your taste buds singing. Paired perfectly with a healthy homemade ranch dressing that is loaded with zippy lemon juice and fresh dill. Let's dig in!

CHIPOTLE CHICKEN SALAD WITH RANCH DRESSING

SERVINGS: 4 | PREP TIME: 15 min | COOK TIME: 16 min
SODIUM PER SERVING: 340 mg

Chicken

1 lb chicken breast, about 4 small or 2 large

1 tbsp honey

½ tbsp smoked paprika

½ tbsp chipotle chili powder

½ tbsp cumin

1 tsp onion salt

½ tsp garlic powder

¼ tsp salt

2 tbsp olive oil

Salad

6 cups spring mix greens

1 cup sweet corn

1 medium avocado, cubed

¾ cup cherry tomatoes, halved

Dressing

½ cup plain Greek yogurt

2 tbsp olive oil

0.25 oz fresh dill, about 2 tbsp chopped

1 tbsp apple cider vinegar

1 tbsp lemon juice

½ tsp onion powder

½ tsp garlic powder

1   Preheat a cast-iron skillet with one tablespoon of olive oil to medium-high heat. Note: you can also grill your chicken or use a non-stick skillet if you prefer.

2   Prepare the chicken breasts. Combine the spices, honey, and remaining one tablespoon of olive oil in a small bowl to form a paste. Spread the spice paste evenly over all sides of each chicken breast.

3   Add seasoned chicken to the hot pan and sear for 6-8 minutes, or until golden. Flip and cover, continue to cook for an additional 6-8 minutes, or until the second side is golden and the chicken reaches an internal temperature of 165F. Remove from heat and allow to cool slightly before slicing into bite-sized cubes or strips.

4   While the chicken is cooking, prepare the salad dressing. Finely chop the dill. In a small mixing bowl, add Greek yogurt, olive oil, dill, onion powder, garlic powder, salt, apple cider vinegar, and lemon juice. Mix together with a fork or whisk until evenly mixed.

5   Assemble four salads. Start by creating a bed of mixed greens in a shallow bowl, top with corn, avocado, tomatoes, chicken, and dressing. Lightly toss the salad to coat everything in the dressing, and enjoy!

Nutrition Facts per Serving

Servings 4 | Calories 384 | Total Fat 23 g | Saturated Fat 4 g

Monounsaturated Fat 13 g | Polyunsaturated Fat 2 g | Trans Fat 0 g

Cholesterol 71 mg | Sodium 340 mg | Total Carbohydrate 18 g

Dietary Fiber 4 g | Sugars 9 g | Protein 28 g

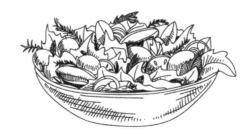

This summer berry salad features juicy strawberries and blue-berries, and a sweet strawberry vinaigrette. In each bite, you will also find creamy goat cheese, crunchy almonds, and punchy red onion. A perfect light lunch!

SUMMER BERRY SALAD WITH STRAW-BERRY VINAIGRETTE

SERVINGS: 4 | PREP TIME: 15 min | SODIUM PER SERVING: 155 mg

Salad

1 cup spinach

6 oz goat cheese

1 cup slivered almonds

¾ cup sliced strawberries

½ cup blueberries

¼ cup red onion

Strawberry Vinaigrette

½ cup strawberries

2 tbsp olive oil

1 tbsp honey

½ tbsp lemon juice

1 tsp balsamic vinegar

1   Prepare the strawberry vinaigrette. Add the strawberries, olive oil, honey, lemon juice, and balsamic vinegar to a blender or food processor. Blend until smooth, about 30 seconds.

2   Prepare the salad mix-ins. Remove the stems from the strawberries, then roughly slice them into bite-sized pieces. Crumble the goat cheese by hand, and finely dice the red onion.

3   Assemble the salad by adding the spinach to a large bowl or plate, top with goat cheese, almonds, strawberries, blueberries, and red onion. Lightly drizzle with the strawberry vinaigrette, toss until evenly coated, and enjoy!

Nutrition Facts per Serving

Servings 4 | Calories 367 | Total Fat 28 g | Saturated Fat 7 g
Monounsaturated Fat 5 g | Polyunsaturated Fat 1 g | Trans Fat 0 g
Cholesterol 38 mg | Sodium 155 mg | Total Carbohydrate 20 g
Dietary Fiber 4 g | Sugars 10 g | Protein 11 g

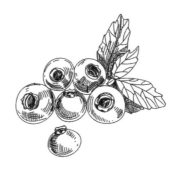

This power greens salad is not your average kale salad. Massaged kale leaves create a soft and tender bed of greens that perfectly carry punchy feta, sweet dried cranberries, nourishing quinoa, and crunchy sunflower seeds. Topped with a sweet and tangy honey mustard dressing, this salad is as delicious as it is healthy!

POWER GREENS SALAD WITH HONEY MUSTARD DRESSING

SERVINGS: 4 | PREP TIME: 10 min | COOK TIME: 15 min
SODIUM PER SERVING: 449 mg

Main Ingredients

1 large bunch of dinosaur kale leaves, about 8-10 leaves

4 oz feta cheese

½ cup dried cranberries, reduced sugar

½ cup quinoa

½ cup water

¼ cup roasted sunflower seeds (preferably unsalted)

1 tbsp olive oil

¼ tsp kosher salt

Honey Mustard Dressing

2 tbsp honey

1 tbsp low-sodium mustard

2 tbsp olive oil

½ tsp apple cider vinegar

1   Add the quinoa and water to a small saucepan with a lid, over high heat. Bring to a boil and stir, reduce heat to low, cover and allow to cook on low for 15 minutes. Remove from heat and fluff quinoa with a fork.

2   Make the honey mustard dressing by combining the honey, mustard, olive oil, and apple cider vinegar. Whisk together until smooth.

3   Prepare the kale. Remove the stems and roughly chop the remaining kale leaves. Add the chopped leaves, olive oil, and salt to a large bowl. Using clean hands, massage the kale by gently kneading the leaves for 1-2 minutes. The kale will appear darker in color and the structure will have softened.

4   Assemble the salad by adding the massaged kale to a large bowl or plate, topping with feta, quinoa, cranberries, sunflower seeds, and the honey mustard dressing. Enjoy!

Nutrition Facts per Serving

Servings 4 | Calories 372 | Total Fat 17 g | Saturated Fat 5 g
Monounsaturated Fat 8 g | Polyunsaturated Fat 2 g | Trans Fat 0 g
Cholesterol 15 mg | Sodium 449 mg | Total Carbohydrate 44 g
Dietary Fiber 10 g | Sugars 15 g | Protein 15 g

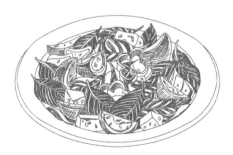

Many soups leave you feeling unsatisfied. Thin, brothy bowls won't keep you fueled and nourished. This shredded chicken tortilla soup is here to change that. Protein-packed chicken breast, fiber-loaded brown rice and vegetables, a smooth and flavorful tomato broth, all topped with a few crunchy tortilla chips, and you have a soup that is filling, delicious, and nutritious!

SHREDDED CHICKEN TORTILLA SOUP

SERVINGS: 4 | PREP TIME: 15 min | COOK TIME: 60 min
SODIUM PER SERVING: 352 mg

16 oz chicken breasts, about 2 large or 4 small

24 oz low-sodium chicken broth

6 oz tomato paste, no salt added

1 large green pepper

2 cups water

3.5 oz green chilis (preferably fresh)

¾ cup corn, fresh or frozen

½ cup brown rice

½ cup sweet yellow onion

3 cloves garlic

1 tbsp cumin

¼ tsp kosher salt

2 oz tortilla chips

1 Preheat a large stockpot with oil to medium heat. Add the chicken breasts and sear for 6-8 minutes, or until lightly golden. Turn and repeat for an additional 6-8 minutes, or until the chicken is cooked through and reaches an internal temperature of 165F.

2 Once the chicken is cooked, use two large forks to shred the chicken. Note: this can be done in the stockpot, or out of the stockpot on a cutting board to avoid burning from hot oil and chicken juices. Simply return the chicken to the stockpot before moving on.

3 Prepare the vegetables by dicing the yellow onion, green peppers, and green chilis, and mincing the garlic.

4 Add the yellow onion and garlic to the pot and allow to sweat for 3-4 minutes, or until slightly translucent.

5 Add the remaining ingredients and stir until well combined. Increase heat to high and bring to a steady boil. Reduce the heat to low, cover, and simmer for 45 minutes, or until the rice is tender.

6 Portion into four bowls, top with tortilla chips, and serve hot!

Nutrition Facts per Serving
Servings 4 | Calories 378 | Total Fat 6 g | Saturated Fat 1 g
Monounsaturated Fat 0 g | Polyunsaturated Fat 0 g | Trans Fat 0 g
Cholesterol 64 mg | Sodium 352 mg | Total Carbohydrate 49 g
Dietary Fiber 6 g | Sugars 11 g | Protein 31 g

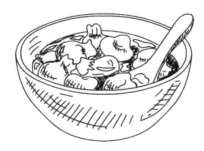

Chili is one of those stews that can carry so many vegetables and mix-ins with ease. Warm and aromatic spices like chili powder and cumin do the heavy lifting while crumbled ground chicken, fiber-filled black beans, tender sweet potatoes, and bell peppers bask in this tomato-based dish.

VEGGIE LOADED CHILI

SERVINGS: 4 | PREP TIME: 15 min | COOK TIME: 45 min
SODIUM PER SERVING: 376 mg

1 lb ground chicken

1 small sweet potato

2 green peppers

½ cup yellow onion

2 cloves garlic

28 oz can crushed tomatoes, no salt added

15 oz can black beans, no salt added

3.5 oz green chilis (preferably fresh)

1 tbsp chili powder

1 tbsp cumin

¼ tsp kosher salt

2 tbsp olive oil

1   Preheat a large stockpot with olive oil to medium heat. Once preheated, add ground chicken. Using a wooden spoon, break up the ground chicken to form a crumble. Stirring occasionally, brown the chicken through, about 6-7 minutes.

2   Prepare the vegetables by mincing garlic, dicing onion, chopping green peppers and green chilis, and cubing sweet potato.

3 Add the garlic, onion, green peppers, green chilis, sweet potato, chili powder, cumin, and kosher salt to the stockpot and stir until the chicken and vegetables are evenly coated in spices.

4 Strain and rinse the black beans. Add the beans, and tomatoes to the stockpot. Reduce heat to medium-low and cover. Allow to simmer for 30-35 minutes, or until sweet potatoes are fork-tender.

5 Portion into four bowls and enjoy!

Nutrition Facts per Serving

Servings 4 | Calories 461 | Total Fat 20 g | Saturated Fat 4 g
Monounsaturated Fat 5 g | Polyunsaturated Fat 1 g | Trans Fat 0 g
Cholesterol 85 mg | Sodium 376 mg | Total Carbohydrate 44 g
Dietary Fiber 11 g | Sugars 12 g | Protein 31 g

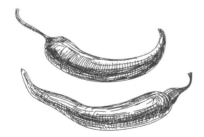

This blended carrot and ginger soup is smooth and creamy and full of flavor. Vibrant turmeric and ginger pack an anti-inflammatory punch, full-fat coconut milk provides a rich and creamy texture, and roasted carrots and sweet potatoes add sweetness and depth of flavor. Top your bowl off with some crispy chickpeas for some plant-powered protein, fiber, and a crunchy change of texture!

BLENDED CARROT GINGER SOUP

SERVINGS: 4 | PREP TIME: 20 min | COOK TIME: 65 min
SODIUM PER SERVING: 276 mg

4 large carrots

2 medium-sized sweet potatoes

15 oz full-fat coconut milk

15 oz can chickpeas (garbanzo beans), no salt added

2 cups vegetable broth, low sodium

2 cups water

½ large sweet yellow onion, about ¾ cup chopped

1 tbsp cumin seeds, whole

1 tsp turmeric powder

½ tsp fresh ground black pepper

¼ tsp sea salt

1 inch fresh ginger, peeled and minced

4 tbsp olive oil

1   Preheat the oven to 400 Fahrenheit.

2   Prepare the crispy chickpeas. Strain and rinse the canned chickpeas, then lightly toss them in one tablespoon of olive oil and sprinkle with sea salt.

3 Add the chickpeas to a rimmed baking sheet lined with parchment paper, and spread to create a single layer. Bake for 50-60 minutes, or until crisp, turning every 20 minutes. Remove from the oven and set aside to cool. Note: monitor the chickpeas closely toward the end to avoid burning. If any chickpeas are burnt, simply remove the individual chickpeas before serving.

4 Prepare carrots and sweet potatoes. Cut the carrots in thirds widthwise, then in half lengthwise. Cut the sweet potatoes into 1/2-inch disks.

5 Toss the carrots and sweet potatoes in two tablespoons of olive oil and spread them in an even layer onto baking sheets. Bake for 25-30 minutes, or until the carrots and potatoes are fork-tender. Note: you may need two separate baking sheets to fit all of the vegetables on a single layer. The chickpeas can continue toasting alongside the vegetables or on a separate rack if your oven has space!

6 Preheat a large stockpot with one tablespoon of olive oil to medium heat.

7 Finely dice the onion and add to the stockpot with cumin seeds. Stirring frequently, sweat onions, and rehydrate cumin until the onions are translucent and the cumin is aromatic, about 2-3 minutes.

8 Add the roasted carrots, sweet potatoes, vegetable broth, coconut milk, turmeric, and black pepper to the stockpot and stir to combine. Increase the heat to medium-high, bring to a boil, and heat through.

9 Remove from the heat, add minced ginger, and blend with an immersion blender until smooth. Note: you can also use a blender or food processor. Allow the soup to cool to just above warm before blending, portion by portion, until the whole batch is smooth.

10 Portion into four bowls, top with crispy chickpeas, and enjoy!

Nutrition Facts per Serving
Servings 4 | Calories 571 | Total Fat 39 g | Saturated Fat 23 g
Monounsaturated Fat 10 g | Polyunsaturated Fat 2 g | Trans Fat 0 g
Cholesterol 0 mg | Sodium 276 mg | Total Carbohydrate 53 g
Dietary Fiber 10 g | Sugars 12 g | Protein 8 g

These Greek grain bowls are loaded with fresh, crisp vegetables, and a zippy dill-infused homemade tzatziki dressing that will be both satisfying and nourishing. Enjoy this vegetarian dish that is packed with protein, fiber, and healthy fats to keep you fueled throughout the day!

GREEK GRAIN BOWL WITH TZATZIKI

SERVINGS: 4 | PREP TIME: 60 min | COOK TIME: 12 min
SODIUM PER SERVING: 145 mg

Toppings

15 oz can chickpeas (garbanzo beans), no salt added

2 small cucumbers

1 cup cherry tomatoes

Couscous

8 oz pearl couscous

1¾ cup water

1 tbsp olive oil

Quick Pickled Onions

1 small shallot

¼ cup apple cider vinegar

1 tbsp raw cane sugar

Pinch of salt

Tzatziki

½ cup plain non-fat Greek yogurt

2 small cucumbers, about ¼ cup shredded and pressed

3 tbsp lemon juice

2 tbsp dill, finely chopped

1 clove garlic, minced

1 tbsp olive oil

1   Start by preparing the quick pickles. Thinly slice the shallot and place it in a small bowl. Submerge with apple cider vinegar, sugar, and salt, and stir. Set aside at room temperature for at least an hour while you assemble the rest of the dish.

2   Prepare the couscous. Preheat a small pot with a lid to medium heat. Add the couscous and toast, stirring frequently until lightly golden, for about 3-4 minutes.

3   Add water and bring to a boil. Reduce heat to low, cover, and simmer for 12 minutes, or until water is absorbed. Fluff with a fork. Note: check directions on the package to verify the cooking time.

4   Prepare the tzatziki. Shred two small cucumbers using a grater or food processor. Using a thin towel or paper towels, press the cucumber by hand to release as much excess moisture as possible.

5   In a medium-sized mixing bowl, combine the Greek yogurt, shredded cucumber, lemon juice, dill, garlic, and olive oil. Stir all ingredients until combined.

6   Prepare the remaining toppings by draining chickpeas, chopping cucumbers, and halving tomatoes.

7   Assemble the bowls by portioning couscous into four bowls, topping with chickpeas, cucumbers, tomatoes, and pickled onions, and drizzle with tzatziki. Enjoy immediately while the couscous is still warm, or refrigerate to enjoy chilled.

Nutrition Facts per Serving

Servings 4 | Calories 521 | Total Fat 12 g | Saturated Fat 3 g
Monounsaturated Fat 5 g | Polyunsaturated Fat 1 g | Trans Fat 0 g
Cholesterol 11 mg | Sodium 145 mg | Total Carbohydrate 83 g
Dietary Fiber 8 g | Sugars 10 g | Protein 18 g

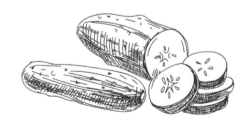

This tofu stir fry bowl features protein-packed tofu, satiating brown rice, and lots of vegetables, all swimming in a robust and flavorful stir fry sauce. This DASH-approved sauce is balanced with lots of flavor elements! Savory low-sodium soy sauce harmoniously works together with a pinch of sugar, garlic, a punch of fresh ginger, a kick of chili paste, and just a hint of sesame oil.

VEGAN TOFU STIR FRY BOWL

SERVINGS: 4 | PREP TIME: 15 min | COOK TIME: 30 min
SODIUM PER SERVING: 427 mg

Main Ingredients

16 oz firm tofu

1 cup brown rice

2 large carrots

2 cups broccoli, chopped

¼ cup white onion

2 tbsp avocado oil

Garnish

¼ cup peanuts, roasted and unsalted

6 green onions, sliced

Stir Fry Sauce

4 tbsp low-sodium soy sauce

⅓ cup water

2 tbsp turbinado sugar

2 cloves garlic, minced

1 inch ginger, about 1 tbsp minced

1 tsp ground chili paste

1 tsp sesame oil

1   Prepare the rice according to the package directions.

2   While the rice is cooking, prepare the tofu. Wrap the tofu in a lint-free cloth
     and place it on a baking sheet with a lip. Press the tofu by placing a cast-iron
     skillet or heavy pan on the tofu and let it sit for at least 5 minutes, periodically
     draining the excess liquid.

3   Prepare the vegetables. While the tofu is pressing, shred carrots, chop
     broccoli, and dice onion.

4   Prepare the stir-fry sauce. In a small bowl, combine the soy sauce, water,
     sugar, ginger, garlic, chili paste, and sesame oil. Whisk together until
     ingredients are thoroughly combined.

5   Preheat a skillet with oil to medium-high heat.

6   Prepare the tofu further by slicing it into small cubes. Add to the hot pan with
     about 1/4-cup of the stir-fry sauce and cook until tofu is golden, about 5-6
     minutes. Remove from the pan and place on a plate lined with a paper towel
     to collect excess moisture.

7   Add the broccoli, onion, and remaining stir-fry sauce to the pan. Stirring
     frequently, cook until the broccoli and onions are tender, for about 7-8
     minutes. Then add the carrots and cook to heat through, about an additional
     minute.

8   Portion the rice into four bowls or plates, top with cooked veggies and sauce,
     tofu, and garnish with peanuts and green onions. Enjoy!

9   When shopping for soy sauce, look for low-sodium soy sauce that has about
     300 mg or less of sodium per tablespoon. Alternatively opt for "coconut
     aminos" which has a similar flavor profile to soy sauce, albeit a little sweeter,
     but with much less sodium.

Nutrition Facts per Serving

Servings 4 | Calories 406 | Total Fat 18 g | Saturated Fat 5 g

Monounsaturated Fat 7 g | Polyunsaturated Fat 2 g | Trans Fat 0 g

Cholesterol 0 mg | Sodium 427 mg | Total Carbohydrate 55 g

Dietary Fiber 8 g | Sugars 12 g | Protein 17 g

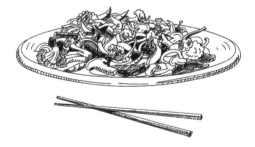

These chickpea salad lettuce wraps are packed with fiber, plant-powered protein, fresh and crisp celery, crunchy carrots, and tender pine nuts. Not to mention, this recipe only takes a few simple steps and not a moment of cooking! This one is as simple as it is delicious. This chickpea salad is also great in whole wheat wraps, on whole-grain toast, or a bed of chopped lettuce as a salad.

CHICKPEA SALAD LETTUCE WRAPS

SERVINGS: 4 | PREP TIME: 10 min | SODIUM PER SERVING: 370 mg

16 butter leaf lettuce leaves, about 1 head (or romaine)

2 x 15 oz cans chickpeas (garbanzo beans), no salt added

6 tbsp mayonnaise (or vegan mayo substitute), low sodium

¼ cup pine nuts

2 tbsp lemon juice

2 stalks celery

2 large carrots, shredded

¼ cup onion, finely diced

1 tsp garlic powder

½ tsp salt

¼ tsp fresh ground black pepper

1 Drain and rinse the chickpeas.

2 Prepare the vegetables by finely chopping the celery, shredding the carrots, and dicing the onion.

3 In a medium-sized mixing bowl, add the chickpeas and roughly mash with a fork. Add mayonnaise, pine nuts, lemon juice, celery, carrots, onion, garlic powder, salt, and pepper. Stir until thoroughly combined.

4 Portion the chickpea salad into individual lettuce leaves, roll, and enjoy. Note: if you're planning to meal prep, store the chickpea salad and lettuce separately and assemble right before eating.

Nutrition Facts per Serving
Servings 4 | Calories 427 | Total Fat 22 g | Saturated Fat 3 g
Monounsaturated Fat 5 g | Polyunsaturated Fat 12 g | Trans Fat 0 g
Cholesterol 9 mg | Sodium 370 mg | Total Carbohydrate 44 g
Dietary Fiber 13 g | Sugars 4 g | Protein 12 g

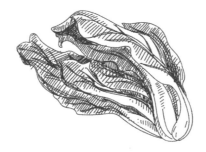

This pesto and roasted veggie pasta is full of fiber-rich vegetables, packed with protein from lentil pasta, and swimming in a fresh and zesty homemade pesto. The homemade pesto features rich olive oil, tender pine nuts, sharp parmesan cheese, zippy lemon, and sweet basil to create a layered sauce that's layered with flavor!

PESTO AND ROASTED VEGGIE PASTA

SERVINGS: 4 | PREP TIME: 10 min | COOK TIME: 25 min
SODIUM PER SERVING: 250 mg

Main Ingredients

8 oz lentil pasta

1 small head broccoli, about 1½ cups chopped

2 small zucchinis

1 tbsp olive oil

Pesto

4 tbsp olive oil

½ lemon, juiced

¼ cup basil, packed

¼ cup spinach, packed

1 clove garlic

2 tbsp parmesan cheese, grated

¼ cup toasted pine nuts

¼ tsp salt

1   Bring a large pot of water to a boil. Add the lentil pasta and cook according to package directions. Strain and rinse the pasta.

2   Preheat the oven to 425 Fahrenheit. Slice the zucchini lengthwise and cut it into half-moons. Roughly chop the broccoli into bite-sized pieces.

3   Toss the zucchini, broccoli, and shallots in 1 tablespoon of olive oil and spread evenly onto a baking sheet. Roast in the preheated oven for 8-10 minutes, or until tender and lightly charred.

4   Prepare the pesto by adding basil, spinach, and pine nuts to a food processor. Pulse until greens are roughly chopped.

5   Add the remaining olive oil, lemon juice, parmesan cheese, garlic, and salt, and continue blending until a loose paste forms.

6   Toss the pasta with pesto and vegetables, portion it into four servings, and enjoy warm!

Nutrition Facts per Serving

Servings 4 | Calories 458 | Total Fat 25 g | Saturated Fat 3 g
Monounsaturated Fat 14 g | Polyunsaturated Fat 4 g | Trans Fat 0 g
Cholesterol 2 mg | Sodium 250 mg | Total Carbohydrate 47 g
Dietary Fiber 15 g | Sugars 3 g | Protein 19 g

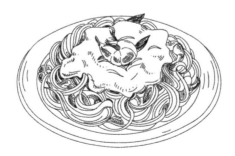

This dish is a plant-based powerhouse and makes tempeh the star of the show. It is loaded with protein and dripping in a sticky honey and garlic glaze that is seriously delicious. Finally, it's rounded out with tender and crispy baked vegetable fries with a simple spice blend that compliments the flavorful tempeh. Dig in!

HONEY & GARLIC TEMPEH

SERVINGS: 4 | PREP TIME: 15 min | COOK TIME: 30 min
SODIUM PER SERVING: 380 mg

Main Ingredients

16 oz tempeh

2 tbsp olive oil, plus more for the pan

4 large cloves garlic, minced

2 tbsp honey

¼ tsp black pepper

¼ tsp kosher salt

Vegetable Fries

6 large carrots

2 medium sweet potatoes

2 tbsp olive oil

½ tsp onion salt

½ tsp smoked paprika

¼ tsp black pepper

1   Preheat the oven to 425 Fahrenheit.

2   Prepare the vegetable fries by cutting them into 1/2-inch thick strips. Start by cutting the carrots and sweet potatoes in half widthwise. Then slice in half lengthwise. Repeat slicing the sections in half lengthwise until you achieve 1/2-inch thick strips. Note: you want your strips roughly the same thickness for best results.

3   Toss the carrots and sweet potato strips in two tablespoons of olive oil, onion salt, paprika, and black pepper until evenly coated.

4   Spread the vegetables in a single layer on a baking sheet and bake for 25 minutes, flipping halfway through, or until tender. Remove from the oven. Note: you want your vegetables to cook in a single layer to avoid soggy fries, use two baking sheets if needed.

5   While the vegetable fries are cooking, prepare the tempeh. Slice the tempeh into strips about 1/2-inch thick.

6   Prepare the honey and garlic glaze by mincing the garlic. In a small bowl, whisk together the garlic, honey, olive oil, black pepper, and kosher salt.

7   In a shallow bowl, add the tempeh and drizzle the glaze over the tempeh. Turn the tempeh to coat it evenly with the glaze.

8   Preheat a large skillet with olive oil to medium heat. Use enough olive oil to lightly coat the pan.

9   Once the pan is preheated, add the tempeh and fry until golden, about 3-4 minutes. Turn, and repeat until the other side is golden.

10 Remove from the pan, portion onto four plated, add vegetable fries, and serve.

Nutrition Facts per Serving
Servings 4 | Calories 530 | Total Fat 25 g | Saturated Fat 2 g
Monounsaturated Fat 10 g | Polyunsaturated Fat 1 g | Trans Fat 0 g
Cholesterol 0 mg | Sodium 380 mg | Total Carbohydrate 42 g
Dietary Fiber 8 g | Sugars 20 g | Protein 23 g

This dish is an updated version of popular comfort food. Each serving delivers nourishing, fiber-filled vegetables and lentils, hidden in warm and cozy flavors. Spaghetti squash carries a lentil-based ragu full of bright tomatoes, tender carrots, crisp celery, and punchy garlic and onions. The perfect DASH comfort food!

VEGAN LENTIL RAGU WITH SPAGHETTI SQUASH

SERVINGS: 4 | PREP TIME: 10 min | COOK TIME: 45 min
SODIUM PER SERVING: 215 mg

4 tbsp olive oil

1 medium spaghetti squash

1 cup red lentils, whole

3 cups low-sodium vegetable broth

2 medium carrots, about 1 cup chopped

1 small shallot

1 stalk celery

2 cloves garlic

2 cups grape tomatoes

½ tsp red pepper flakes

¼ cup white wine, dry

1   Preheat the oven to 400 Fahrenheit.

2   Prepare the squash by slicing it in half and spooning out the seeds and innards. Lightly drizzle the squash with two tablespoons of olive oil and bake, skin side down for 40 minutes, or until fork-tender.

3   While the spaghetti squash is cooking, preheat a skillet with the remaining olive oil to medium heat.

4   Prepare the vegetables. Dice carrots, shallot, and celery, and mince garlic.

5   Add the shallots, celery, carrots, and garlic to the pan and cook until aromatic and shallots appear translucent, about 3-4 minutes.

6   Add the tomatoes, red pepper flakes, and white wine. Bring to a boil, reduce to a steady simmer.

7   Allow to simmer and cook, stirring occasionally until the wine has reduced in volume by about half.

8   Add the lentils and broth, and bring to a boil. Reduce heat to low, cover, and allow to simmer for 15-20 minutes, until lentils are tender and the tomatoes have burst. Note: if you use split lentils, refer to the package instructions for cooking time.

9   Remove the spaghetti squash from the oven and pull the spaghetti squash from the skin with a fork until all of it is released.

10 Plate the squash onto four plates, add lentil ragu, and enjoy warm!

Nutrition Facts per Serving
Servings 4 | Calories 312 | Total Fat 14 g | Saturated Fat 2 g
Monounsaturated Fat 10 g | Polyunsaturated Fat 2 g | Trans Fat 0 g
Cholesterol 0 mg | Sodium 215 mg | Total Carbohydrate 36 g
Dietary Fiber 12 g | Sugars 14 g | Protein 8 g

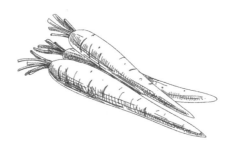

This vegan Thai coconut curry features some serious flavor. This dish combines a rich and creamy coconut milk broth, aromatic red curry paste, spicy ginger, and sweet and juicy mango for a complex and unique experience. Enjoy this dish over rice, or as a soup. Either way, you're in for a treat!

VEGAN THAI COCONUT CURRY

SERVINGS: 4 | PREP TIME: 10 min | COOK TIME: 20 min
SODIUM PER SERVING: 377 mg

8 oz tempeh

15 oz can chickpeas (garbanzo beans), no salt added

15 oz can full-fat coconut milk

1 cup water

2 bell peppers, red or orange

1 medium-sized mango

2 tbsp coconut oil

2 tbsp red curry paste

2 cloves garlic

1 inch ginger

1 small shallot

¼ tsp salt

Thai basil for garnish

1   Preheat a large saucepan with coconut oil to medium heat.

2   Prepare the ingredients. Strain and rinse chickpeas, crumble tempeh by hand into bite-sized pieces, remove stems and seeds from bell peppers and slice into 1/2-inch strips, remove skin and pit from mango and slice into cubes, dice shallot, and mince ginger.

3 Once the skillet is preheated, add the shallots, ginger, and garlic and cook until fragrant, about 2-3 minutes.

4 Add the tempeh, curry paste, and salt. Cook, stirring frequently until tempeh is golden, about 4-5 minutes.

5 Add the chickpeas, coconut milk, water, peppers, and mango, and stir. Bring mixture to a boil, then reduce heat to a simmer, cover, and cook until peppers are tender, about 6-8 minutes.

6 Portion into four bowls, top with fresh Thai basil, and enjoy warm. Optional: serve over brown rice.

Nutrition Facts per Serving

Servings 4 | Calories 523 | Total Fat 30 g | Saturated Fat 22 g

Monounsaturated Fat 0 g | Polyunsaturated Fat 0 g | Trans Fat 0 g

Cholesterol 0 mg | Sodium 377 mg | Total Carbohydrate 41 g

Dietary Fiber 8 g | Sugars 11 g | Protein 19 g

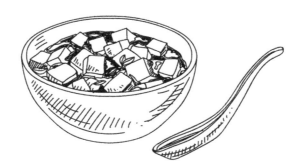

This seared sirloin with chimichurri is full of lean protein and fresh flavors. Chimichurri is packed with leafy herbs and punchy onions, jalapeno, and garlic to add brightness to this savory protein and roasted asparagus. Get ready for a DASH-friendly classic!

SEARED SIRLOIN WITH CHIMICHURRI SAUCE

SERVINGS: 4 | PREP TIME: 45 min | COOK TIME: 20 min
SODIUM PER SERVING: 231 mg

Main Ingredients

16 oz sirloin, 4 small steaks

1 bunch asparagus

½ large red onion

2 tbsp olive oil

Chimichurri

½ medium shallot

½ jalapeño

3 garlic cloves

⅓ cup red wine vinegar

½ tsp kosher salt

¼ cup cilantro, packed

½ cup parsley, packed

6 tbsp extra-virgin olive oil

1 Preheat the oven to 425 Fahrenheit.

2   Prepare the chimichurri. Finely slice the shallot, removing the papery skin and roots, slice the garlic cloves, and finely dice the jalapeno, removing seeds and ribs. Add the shallot, garlic, and jalapeno to a medium-sized bowl, submerge in vinegar and salt, and set aside.

3   Chop the cilantro and parsley, discarding the stems. Add the cilantro, parsley, and olive oil to the vinegar mixture and stir to combine.

4   On a large plate, spoon about half of the chimichurri mixture onto the steaks, gently spreading the mixture evenly over the surface of each steak. Refrigerate and marinate for at least 30 minutes, and up to overnight.

5   Meanwhile, prepare the vegetables by slicing off the stems of the asparagus and chopping the red onion into strips. Lightly toss in oil and spread into an even layer on a baking sheet. Bake for 8-10 minutes, or until asparagus is fork-tender.

6   Preheat a medium-sized skillet, lightly oiled to medium-high heat. Once the skillet is hot, sear each steak to the desired doneness. For medium-rare steaks, sear for about 5 minutes per side. Remove the steaks from the heat and rest for 5-10 minutes before slicing thinly and serving.

7   Plate the steaks with asparagus, onions, and drizzle everything with the remaining chimichurri. Enjoy!

Nutrition Facts per Serving

Servings 4 | Calories 405 | Total Fat 31 g | Saturated Fat 10 g

Monounsaturated Fat 10 g | Polyunsaturated Fat 14 g

Trans Fat 0 g | Cholesterol 72 mg | Sodium 231 mg

Total Carbohydrate 7 g | Dietary Fiber 2 g | Sugars 3 g | Protein 25 g

These sirloin & veggie kebabs may be simple, but what makes them extraordinary is a thick and gut-friendly garlic yogurt dip that is so good, you could practically eat it by the spoonful. Rich and creamy with a punch of freshly minced garlic to add just the right burst of flavor to every bite. So, fire up your grill, and let's get cooking!

SIRLOIN & VEGGIE KEBABS WITH GARLIC YOGURT DIP

SERVINGS: 4 | PREP TIME: 10 min | COOK TIME: 12 min
SODIUM PER SERVING: 182 mg

Main Ingredients

16 oz sirloin, 4 small steaks

½ tsp kosher salt

½ tsp black pepper

½ large red onion

1 medium-sized zucchini

1 medium-sized summer squash

Olive oil spray

Yogurt Dip

½ cup plain Greek yogurt

3 tbsp olive oil

3 cloves garlic

¼ tsp garlic powder

¼ tsp onion powder

¼ tsp sea salt

1   Preheat your grill to medium heat, about 450 Fahrenheit.

2 Prepare the kebabs by cutting the steak into even, bite-sized cubes. Chop the onions into large chunks, and slice the zucchini and summer squash into 2-inch thick disks.

3 Assemble the kebabs. Using metal skewers, puncture the steak through the center, add onion by poking through the center, add zucchini and summer squash by puncturing through the skin on both sides. Repeat until skewers are even. Note: if you choose to use wooden skewers, be sure to soak them in water overnight to prevent burning.

4 Lightly spray the kebabs with olive oil and sprinkle with salt and pepper.

5 Prepare the garlic yogurt dip. Whisk together the yogurt, olive oil, minced garlic, garlic powder, onion powder, and sea salt until smooth and creamy.

6 Place on the grill and grill for about 2 minutes per side, or until the steak is evenly charred and cooked to desired doneness. Note: if you prefer your steak on the rare side, you may want to prepare separate steak kebabs and vegetable kebabs to ensure the vegetables have enough time to cook and reach desired tenderness.

7 Portion onto four plates and enjoy!

Nutrition Facts per Serving
Servings 4 | Calories 328 | Total Fat 17 g | Saturated Fat 4 g
Monounsaturated Fat 10 g | Polyunsaturated Fat 1 g | Trans Fat 0 g
Cholesterol 88 mg | Sodium 182 mg | Total Carbohydrate 6 g
Dietary Fiber 1 g | Sugars 3 g | Protein 39 g

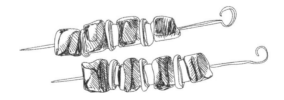

This pork tenderloin sheet pan meal is perfect for any weeknight. Tender pork tenderloin, potato wedges, and sweet carrots are smothered in a creamy, sweet, and punchy homemade honey mustard sauce. This meal requires just a little bit of prep, then you are free to leave it in the oven to bathe in this simple sauce and work its magic.

HONEY MUSTARD PORK TENDERLOIN

SERVINGS: 4 | PREP TIME: 5 min | COOK TIME: 35 min
SODIUM PER SERVING: 433 mg

1 lb pork tenderloin

5 medium carrots

2 medium Yukon gold potatoes

¼ cup low-sodium mustard

¼ cup olive oil

¼ cup honey

1   Preheat the oven to 400 Fahrenheit.

2   Whisk together the mustard, olive oil, and honey until smooth.

3   Carefully slice away any excess fat from the tenderloin and discard, slice the potatoes into wedges, and cut the carrots into strips.

4   Place everything on a large baking sheet and cover it in honey mustard. Note: for easy clean-up, line the baking sheet with foil, then rinse and recycle when done!

5   Bake for 25-35 minutes, or until the tenderloin reaches 145F in the center, and the vegetables are fork-tender.

6   Rest for 5-10 minutes before slicing, portioning into four servings, and enjoy!

Nutrition Facts per Serving

Servings 4 | Calories 479 | Total Fat 18 g | Saturated Fat 3 g
Monounsaturated Fat 11 g | Polyunsaturated Fat 2 g | Trans Fat 0 g
Cholesterol 83 mg | Sodium 433 mg | Total Carbohydrate 40 g
Dietary Fiber 6 g | Sugars 25 g | Protein 32 g

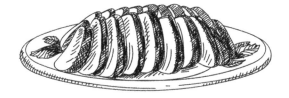

Dig into savory pork chops with a sweet brown sugar rub and warm cinnamon apples. Paired with tender sweet potatoes that will melt in your mouth. This meal is filling and delicious, with less than 400 calories per serving. A must-add to your weeknight rotation!

PORK CHOPS WITH SWEET CINNAMON APPLES

SERVINGS: 4 | PREP TIME: 15 min | COOK TIME: 50 min
SODIUM PER SERVING: 110 mg

Pork Chops

16 oz pork chops, about 4 small chops

2 tbsp olive oil

2 tbsp brown sugar, packed

1 tsp garlic powder

Cinnamon Apples

3 small apples

2 tbsp maple syrup

1 tsp cinnamon

Sweet Potatoes

2 medium-sized sweet potatoes

½ cup low-sodium vegetable broth

2 tbsp unsalted butter

1 tbsp sage, finely chopped and packed

½ tsp pepper

1 Preheat the oven to 425 Fahrenheit.

2   Prepare the sweet potatoes. Slice the sweet potatoes into thick disks, about 2-inches thick. Melt the butter, and whisk in sage and pepper. Toss the sweet potatoes with the butter and sage mixture until evenly coated.

3   Arrange the sweet potatoes into a single layer on a rimmed baking sheet and bake for 15 minutes.

4   While the sweet potatoes are cooking, prepare the cinnamon apples. Cube the apples, removing the seeds and stems. Add apples, maple syrup, and cinnamon to a small saucepan over medium-low heat. Allow to simmer, keep covered until soft and tender, about 15 minutes. Stir the apples occasionally to make sure nothing is sticking. Add a splash of water if needed. Remove from the heat once they are cooked and set aside.

5   Meanwhile, prepare the pork chops by whisking together the olive oil, brown sugar, and garlic powder. Pat the pork chops dry with a paper towel and evenly spoon the rub onto all sides of each pork chop. Place on a baking sheet.

6   After the sweet potatoes have been baking for 15 minutes, place the pork chops in the oven and flip the sweet potatoes.

7   Allow the sweet potatoes and pork chops to bake for 20 minutes, or until the pork chops reach an internal temperature of 145 Fahrenheit. Remove the pork chops from the oven and allow to rest.

8   Carefully add vegetable broth to the rimmed baking sheet with the sweet potatoes, and allow to bake for another 15 minutes, or until the broth is fully absorbed. Remove from the oven and allow to cool before handling.

9   Plate the pork chops, top with cinnamon apples, and portion sweet potatoes onto four plates, and enjoy!

Nutrition Facts per Serving
Servings 4 | Calories 406 | Total Fat 17 g | Saturated Fat 6 g
Monounsaturated Fat 6 g | Polyunsaturated Fat 1 g | Trans Fat 0 g
Cholesterol 70 mg | Sodium 110 mg | Total Carbohydrate 43 g
Dietary Fiber 5 g | Sugars 28 g | Protein 24 g

ABOUT THE AUTHOR

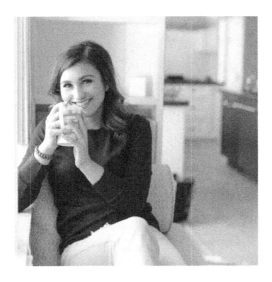

Elaine Summers is a Registered Dietitian Nutritionist (RDN) with a master's degree in Nutrition and Dietetics.

As someone who had struggled with her health and weight throughout childhood, Elaine has made it her life's goal to become a serial researcher and expert nutritionist. She has helped tens of thousands of clients around the world who went through similar struggles to now live longer, healthier, and happier lives.

Elaine has also spent several years as a research and development chef in the fine dining industry, including restaurants, hotels, and even a gourmet chocolate boutique. As a result, she has a keen eye for developing recipes that are not only healthy and nutritious, but also satisfy the deepest cravings.

In addition to sharing her knowledge through her book series, Elaine is a frequent contributor to various established blogs, podcasts, and online publications. She enjoys spending her free time in her kitchen, developing healthy recipes for her loving family.

DASH Food Group Table

	Serving Sizes	Whole Grains
Whole Grains	Serving Sizes 1/2 cup cooked whole grains or pasta. 1 ounce dry cereal or crackers. 1 slice of bread. 1 small tortilla.	**Whole Grains** Amaranth, barley, brown rice, buckwheat, bulgur, corn kernels, couscous, farro, freekeh, kaniwa, kamut, millet, oats, orzo, psyllium, quinoa, rye, sorghum, spelt, teff, triticale, wheat, wild rice. **Processed Whole Grains** Bagels, bread, cereal, corn tortillas, crackers, English muffins, pasta, popcorn, rolls.
Vegetables	Serving Sizes 1 cup raw leafy greens. 1/2 cup cut, raw or cooked vegetables. 1/2 cup vegetable juice.	**Cruciferous Vegetables** Bok choy, broccoli, Brussels sprouts, cauliflower, green cabbage, red cabbage, radish, savoy cabbage, turnips. **Leafy Greens** Arugula, beet greens, bibb lettuce, broccoli rabe (rapini), butter lettuce, chicory, collard greens, dandelion greens, endive, iceberg lettuce, kale, mustard greens, Napa cabbage, red leaf lettuce, romaine lettuce, spinach, Swiss chard, turnip greens, watercress. **Legumes** Alfalfa, green beans, lentils, snow peas, sugar snap peas.

Vegetables		**Root Vegetables** Arrowroot, beets, carrots, cassava. celery root, daikon, fennel, ginger, horseradish, jicama, kohlrabi, lotus root, parsnip, red onion, red potato, Russet potato, rutabaga, shallots, sweet onion, sweet potato, taro, white onion, yam root, yellow onion. **Squash and Gourds** Acorn, amber, ambercup, arikara, autumn cup, banana squash, bitter melon, buttercup, butternut, calabaza, carnival, chayote, crookneck, cucumber, cushaw, delicata, gem, gold nugget, hubbard, Jarrahdale pumpkin, kabocha, lakota, mooregold, patty pan, pumpkin, red kuri, spaghetti squash, sugar loaf, sweet dumpling, turban, yellow squash, yellow zucchini, zucchini. **Others** Artichoke. asparagus, bell pepper, celery, corn on the cob, eggplant, heart of palm, leeks, mushroom, okra, radicchio, tomatillo, tomato.

Fruit	**Serving Sizes** 1/2 cup fresh, frozen, or canned fruit. 1 medium-sized fruit. 1/4 cup dried fruit. 1/2 cup fruit juice.	**Berries** Blackberries, blueberries, boysenberries, cranberries, elderberries, gooseberries, loganberries, mulberries, raspberries, strawberries. **Citrus** Clementine, grapefruit, kumquat, lemon, lime, mandarin oranges, nectarine, orange, pomelo, tangerine. **Tropical** Avocado, banana, breadfruit, coconut meat, custard apple, dragon fruit, durian, fig, guava, jackfruit, kiwi, longan, lychee, mangoes, mangosteen, papaya, passion fruit, persimmon, pineapple, pomegranate seeds, rambutan, soursop, starfruit, sugar-apple, watermelon. **Others** Apples, apricots, Asian pear, blackcurrant, cantaloupe, cherimoya, cherries, dried fruit (no added sugar), grapes, honeydew, Medjool dates, olives, peaches, pears, plantain, plums, prickly pear, prunes, raisins (no added sugar).

Nuts, Seeds, Beans, Peas	**Serving Sizes** 1/2 cup cooked legumes. 2 tablespoons nut butter. 1/3 cup or 1 1/2 ounces nuts. 2 tablespoons or 1/2 ounce seeds. 1/2 cup tofu.	**Nuts** Almond, almond butter, Brazil nut, cashew, cashew butter, chestnut, hazelnut, macadamia, Marcona almond, peanut, peanut butter, pecan, pili nut, pine nut, pistachio, tiger nut, walnut. **Seeds** Chia, flax, hemp, jackfruit seed, papaya seed, poppy, pumpkin seed, sesame, sunflower, squash seed, watermelon seed. **Beans** Adzuki, black, black-eyed, cannellini, chickpea (garbanzo), cranberry, edamame, fava, Great Northern, kidney, lima, mung, pinto, navy, white, yellow, soybeans, and tofu. **Peas** English peas, green peas, split peas.
Fats and Oils	**Serving Sizes** 1 teaspoon oil or other liquid fats. 1 teaspoon margarine or butter. 2 tablespoons low-fat salad dressing (or 1 tbsp regular dressing).	**Heart-Healthy Fats** Margarine (soft or liquid), salad dressings, sunflower seed butter, vegetable oil spread. **Oils** Avocado, canola, olive, peanut, safflower, soybean, walnut.

Dairy	**Serving Sizes** 1 cup milk. 1 cup yogurt. 1 1/2 ounces cheese.	**Dairy** Low-fat and fat-free plain milk, yogurt (no added sugar), and cheese. **Plant-Based** Calcium-fortified plant-based milk and yogurt (no added sugar). Plant-based made from almond, cashew, hemp, macadamia, oat, pea, or soy.
Meat, Poultry and Fish	**Serving Sizes** 1 ounce cooked meat, poultry, or fish. 1 egg or 2 egg whites.	**Meats** Canadian bacon, beef loin, beef round, ground beef (at least 90% lean), lamb leg, lamb loin, lamb rib, lamb shoulder, pork loin, pork round, veal rib, veal shoulder, venison, wild game. **Poultry** Chicken breast (skinless), egg, ground chicken, ground turkey, turkey. **Fish** Albacore tuna, flounder, herring, mackerel, salmon, sardines, tilapia, trout.

US Standard to Metric Conversions

Cooking Temperatures

Fahrenheit	Celsius	Gas Mark
145° F	63° C	-
160° F	71° C	-
165° F	74° C	-
250° F	120° C	1/2
275° F	140° C	1
300° F	150° C	2
325° F	160° C	3
350° F	180° C	4
375° F	190° C	5
400° F	200° C	6
425° F	220° C	7
450° F	230° C	8
475° F	250° C	9

Ingredients by Weight

Ounces	Pounds	Grams
1/4 oz	-	7 g
1/2 oz	-	15 g
1 oz	1/16 lb	30 g
2 oz	1/8 lb	55 g
4 oz	1/4 lb	115 g
6 oz	3/8 lb	170 g
8 oz	1/2 lb	230 g
12 oz	3/4 lb	340 g
15 oz	0.9 lb	430 g

16 oz	1 lb	450 g
28 oz	1.75 lb	800 g

Ingredients by Volume

Spoons	Cups	Fluid Ounces	Milliliters
1/8 tsp	-	-	0.625 ml
1/4 tsp	-	-	1.25 ml
1/2 tsp	-	-	2.5 ml
1 tsp	-	-	5 ml
1/2 tbsp	-	-	7.5 ml
1 tbsp	1/16 cup	1/2 fl oz	15 ml
2 tbsp	1/8 cup	1 fl oz	30 ml
4 tbsp	1/4 cup	2 fl oz	60 ml
-	1/3 cup	3 fl oz	80 ml
8 tbsp	1/2 cup	4 fl oz	120 ml
-	2/3 cup	5 fl oz	160 ml
12 tbsp	3/4 cup	6 fl oz	180 ml
16 tbsp	1 cup	8 fl oz	240 ml
1 pint	2 cups	16 fl oz	480 ml
1.5 pint	3 cups	24 fl oz	710 ml
1 quart	4 cups	32 fl oz	960 ml

Ingredients by Length

Inches	Feet	Centimeters
1 in	-	2.5 cm
6 in	1/2 ft	15 cm
12 in	1 ft	30 cm
24 in	2 ft	60 cm

References

1. Xenaki, Niovi et al. "Impact of a stress management program on weight loss, mental health and lifestyle in adults with obesity: a randomized controlled trial." Journal of molecular biochemistry vol. 7,2 (2018): 78-84.

2. "Monitoring Your Blood Pressure at Home." www.heart.org/en/health-topics/high-blood-pressure/understanding-blood-pressure-readings/monitoring-your-blood-pressure-at-home.

3. National Institutes of Health. "Your Guide to Lowering Your Blood Pressure with DASH." NIH Publication No. 06-4082, 2006.

4. Challa, Ameer et al. "DASH Diet to Stop Hypertension." StatPearls Publishing, 2021.

5. "Department of Health and Human Services, Facts & Statistics of Physical Activity." www.hhs.gov/fitness/resource-center/facts-and-statistics/index.html

6. Centers for Disease Control and Prevention. "State Indicator Report on Fruits and Vegetables." U.S. Department of Health and Human Services, 2018.

7. Kyrou, Randeva et al. "Clinical Problems Caused by Obesity." MDText.com, Inc., South Dartmouth (MA), 2018.

8. "Centers for Disease Control and Prevention, High blood pressure frequently asked questions." www.cdc.gov/bloodpressure/facts.htm

9. "National Institutes of Health, DASH ranked Best Diet Overall for eighth year in a row by U.S. News and World Report." www.nih.gov/news-events/news-releases/dash-ranked-best-diet-overall-eighth-year-row-us-news-world-report

10. Sacks, Svetkey et al. "Effects on blood pressure of reduced dietary sodium and the dietary approaches to stop hypertension (DASH) diet." The New England Journal of Medicine 344(1), 3-10 (2001).

11. Centers for Disease Control and Prevention. "Underlying Cause of Death, 1999–2018." CDC Online Database. Atlanta, GA, 2018.

12. Appel, Moore et al. "A clinical trial of the effects of dietary patterns on blood pressure." The New England Journal of Medicine, 336(16), 1117–1124 (1997).

13. Al-Solaiman, Jesri et al. "DASH lowers blood pressure in obese hypertensives beyond potassium, magnesium and fiber." Journal of Human Hypertension, 24(4), 237-246, 2009.

14. Center for Food Safety and Applied Nutrition. " Science and Our Food Supply: Using the Nutrition Facts Label to Make Healthy Food Choices." Food and Drug Administration, 2017.

15. Whelton, Paul K et al. "Sodium, blood pressure, and cardiovascular disease: further evidence supporting the American Heart Association sodium reduction recommendations." Circulation vol. 126,24 (2012): 2880-9.

16. Whelton, Paul K. "Urinary sodium and cardiovascular disease risk: informing guidelines for sodium consumption." JAMA vol. 306,20 (2011): 2262-4.

17. "Harvard School of Public Health, The Nutrition Source - Salt and Sodium" https://www.hsph.harvard.edu/nutritionsource/salt-and-sodium/

18. Duyff. "Complete Food & Nutrition Guide." New York Academy of Nutrition and Dietetics, 2017.

19. Gropper & Smith. "Advanced Nutrition and Human Metabolism." Cengage Learning, 2013.
20. He, Feng J, and Graham A MacGregor. "Beneficial effects of potassium on human health." Physiologia plantarum vol. 133,4 (2008): 725-35.
21. McDonough, Alicia A, and Mien T X Nguyen. "How does potassium supplementation lower blood pressure?." American journal of physiology. Renal physiology vol. 302,9 (2012): F1224-5.
22. "National Institute of Health, Potassium Fact Sheet for Health Professionals" https://ods.od.nih.gov/factsheets/Potassium-HealthProfessional/
23. Gröber, Uwe et al. "Magnesium in Prevention and Therapy." Nutrients vol. 7,9 8199-226. 23 Sep 2015.
24. Zhang, Xi et al. "Effects of Magnesium Supplementation on Blood Pressure: A Meta-Analysis of Randomized Double-Blind Placebo-Controlled Trials." Hypertension vol. 68,2 (2016): 324-33.
25. Villa-Etchegoyen, Cecilia et al. "Mechanisms Involved in the Relationship between Low Calcium Intake and High Blood Pressure." Nutrients vol. 11,5 1112. May. 2019.
26. Kim, Mi-Hyun et al. "Daily calcium intake and its relation to blood pressure, blood lipids, and oxidative stress biomarkers in hypertensive and normotensive subjects." Nutrition research and practice vol. 6,5. 2012.
27. Margolis, Karen L et al. "Effect of calcium and vitamin D supplementation on blood pressure: the Women's Health Initiative Randomized Trial." Hypertension vol. 52,5 (2008): 847-55.
28. Soliman, Ghada A. "Dietary Fiber, Atherosclerosis, and Cardiovascular Disease." Nutrients vol. 11,5 1155. 23 May. 2019.
29. Surampudi, Prasanth et al. "Lipid Lowering with Soluble Dietary Fiber." Current atherosclerosis reports vol. 18,12 (2016): 75.
30. "Harvard School of Public Health, The Nutrition Source - Whole Grains." https://www.hsph.harvard.edu/nutritionsource/what-should-you-eat/whole-grains.
31. Papanikolaou, Jones et al. "Several grain dietary patterns are associated with better diet quality and improved shortfall nutrient intakes in US children and adolescents: a study focusing on the 2015–2020 Dietary Guidelines for Americans." Nutr J 16, 13 (2017).
32. "National Heart Lung and Blood Institute, DASH Eating Plan." www.nhlbi.nih.gov/health-topics/dash-eating-plan.
33. Slavin, Joanne L, and Beate Lloyd. "Health benefits of fruits and vegetables." Advances in nutrition (Bethesda, Md.) vol. 3,4 506-16. 1 Jul. 2012.
34. McGrane, Mary M et al. "Dairy Consumption, Blood Pressure, and Risk of Hypertension: An Evidence-Based Review of Recent Literature." Current cardiovascular risk reports vol. 5,4, 2011.
35. Wright K. C. "The Coup in the Dairy Aisle." Today's Dietitian, 20(9), 28 (2018).
36. Schönfeldt, Pretorius et al. " The impact of animal source food products on human nutrition and health." South African Journal of Animal Science Vol. 43 No. 3 (2013).
37. Elmadfa & Meyer. "Animal Proteins as Important Contributors to a Healthy Human Diet." Annual Review of Animal Biosciences 5(1), 2016.

38. "U.S. Department of Agriculture, What's Your Beef – Prime, Choice or Select?" https://www.usda.gov/media/blog/2013/01/28/whats-your-beef-prime-choice-or-select

39. Howard, B V et al. "LDL cholesterol as a strong predictor of coronary heart disease in diabetic individuals with insulin resistance and low LDL: The Strong Heart Study." Arteriosclerosis, thrombosis, and vascular biology vol. 20,3 (2000).

40. Carson, Lichtenstein et al. " Dietary Cholesterol and Cardiovascular Risk: A Science Advisory from the American Heart Association." AHA Journals Circulation. 2020, 141, e39–e53.

41. Frankenfield, David et al. "Comparison of predictive equations for resting metabolic rate in healthy nonobese and obese adults: a systematic review." Journal of the American Dietetic Association vol. 105,5 (2005): 775-89.

42. Matthews. "Bigger Leaner Stronger: The Simple Science of Building the Ultimate Male Body." Oculus Publishers; 3rd edition, 2019.

43. Matthews. "Thinner Leaner Stronger: The Simple Science of Building the Ultimate Female Body." Oculus Publishers; 3rd edition, 2019.

44. Huovinen, Heikki T et al. "Body composition and power performance improved after weight reduction in male athletes without hampering hormonal balance." Journal of strength and conditioning research vol. 29,1 (2015): 29-36.

45. "WebMD, Selected ACE Inhibitors / Potassium Supplements Interactions." https://www.webmd.com/drugs/2/drug-676-674/potassium-chloride-oral/potassium-extended-release-oral/details/list-interaction-details/dmid-3138/dmtitle-potassium-supplements-selected-ace-inhibitors/intrtype-drug.

46. Doorenbos, C J, and C G Vermeij. "Danger of salt substitutes that contain potassium in patients with renal failure." BMJ (Clinical research ed.) vol. 326,7379 (2003): 35-6.

47. U.S. Department of Agriculture, Agricultural Research Service. "National Nutrient Database for Standard Reference, Release 25, current manufacturers' data."

48. Mariotti, François, and Christopher D Gardner. "Dietary Protein and Amino Acids in Vegetarian Diets-A Review." Nutrients vol. 11,11 2661. 4 Nov. 2019.

49. Mangels, Ann Reed. "Bone nutrients for vegetarians." The American journal of clinical nutrition vol. 100 Suppl 1 (2014).

50. Bacon, Simon L et al. "Effects of exercise, diet and weight loss on high blood pressure." Sports medicine (Auckland, N.Z.) vol. 34,5 (2004).

51. Neter, Stam et al. "Influence of Weight Reduction on Blood Pressure, A Meta-Analysis of Randomized Controlled Trials." AHA Journal Hypertension. 2003;42:878–884.

52. Brown, Joshua D et al. "Effects on cardiovascular risk factors of weight losses limited to 5-10." Translational behavioral medicine vol. 6,3 (2016).

53. Poobalan, A et al. "Effects of weight loss in overweight/obese individuals and long-term lipid outcomes--a systematic review." Journal of the International Association for the Study of Obesity vol. 5,1 (2004).

54. Virdis, Giannarelli et al. "Cigarette smoking and hypertension." Current Pharmaceutical Design, 16(23), 2518-25, (2010).

55. Nelms, Sucher et al. "Nutrition Therapy and Pathophysiology, 3e." Boston Cengage Learning, 2016.

56. Harris, C. "Mindful Eating - Studies Show This Concept Can Help Clients Lose Weight and Better Manage Chronic Disease." Today's Dietitian, 15(3), 42, (2013).
57. May, M. "Eat What You Love, Love What You Eat." Am I Hungry Publishing, 2017.
58. Kok, P et al. "The value and limitations of the body mass index (BMI) in the assessment of the health risks of overweight and obesity." Nederlands tijdschrift voor geneeskunde vol. 148,48 (2004).
59. "Centers for Disease Control and Prevention, What is BMI." www.cdc.gov/healthyweight/assessing/bmi/adult_bmi/index.html
60. Stern, M P, and S M Haffner. "Body fat distribution and hyperinsulinemia as risk factors for diabetes and cardiovascular disease." Arteriosclerosis (Dallas, Tex.) vol. 6,2 (1986).
61. Livingston, Edward H. "Lower body subcutaneous fat accumulation and diabetes mellitus risk." Surgery for obesity and related diseases: Official journal of the American Society for Bariatric Surgery vol. 2,3 (2006).
62. "National Heart, Lung, and Blood Institute, Assessing Your Weight and Health Risk." https://www.nhlbi.nih.gov/health/educational/lose_wt/risk.htm
63. Boyle & Morris. "Community Nutrition in Action, 2e." Wadsworth Publishing Company, 1999.
64. Walia, B N et al. "Reliability of skinfold calipers as a tool for measuring body fat in human beings." The Indian journal of medical research vol. 96 (1992): 255-7.
65. Graybeal, Austin J et al. "Body Composition Assessment in Male and Female Bodybuilders: A 4-Compartment Model Comparison of Dual-Energy X-Ray Absorptiometry and Impedance-Based Devices." Journal of strength and conditioning research vol. 34,6 (2020): 1676-1689.
66. Thomas, Diana M et al. "Effect of dietary adherence on the body weight plateau: a mathematical model incorporating intermittent compliance with energy intake prescription." The American journal of clinical nutrition vol. 100,3 (2014).
67. Escott-Stump. "Nutrition & Diagnosis-Related Care, 8e." Wolters Kluwer, 2015.
68. Swain, McCarron et al. "Characteristics of the diet patterns tested in the optimal macronutrient intake trial to prevent heart disease (OmniHeart): Options for a heart-healthy diet." Journal of the Academy of Nutrition and Dietetics, 108(2), 257-265, (2008).
69. "American Diabetes Association, Glycemic index and diabetes." http://www.diabetes.org/food-and-fitness/food/what-can-i-eat/understanding-carbohydrates/glycemic-index-and-diabetes.html
70. Sacks, Frank M et al. "Effects of high vs low glycemic index of dietary carbohydrate on cardiovascular disease risk factors and insulin sensitivity: the OmniCarb randomized clinical trial." JAMA vol. 312,23 (2014).
71. Ball, Shauna D et al. "Prolongation of satiety after low versus moderately high glycemic index meals in obese adolescents." Pediatrics vol. 111,3 (2003).
72. McKeown, Nicola M et al. "Carbohydrate nutrition, insulin resistance, and the prevalence of the metabolic syndrome in the Framingham Offspring Cohort." Diabetes care vol. 27,2 (2004).
73. Appel, Champagne et al. "Effects of comprehensive lifestyle modification on blood pressure control: Main results of the PREMIER clinical trial." The Journal of the American Medical Association, 289(16), 2083-2093, (2003).

74. Hall & Guyton. "Guyton and Hall Textbook of Medical Physiology, 12th ed." Saunders Elsevier, (2011).
75. Joyner, Michael J, and Darren P Casey. "Regulation of increased blood flow (hyperemia) to muscles during exercise: a hierarchy of competing physiological needs." Physiological reviews vol. 95,2 (2015).
76. Fountain & Lappin. "Physiology, Renin Angiotensin System." StatPearls Publishing, 2019.
77. Wittner, M et al. "How do loop diuretics act?." Drugs vol. 41 Suppl 3 (1991): 1-13.
78. Herman, Padala et al. "Angiotensin Converting Enzyme Inhibitors (ACEI)." StatPearls Publishing, 2020.
79. Prichard, B N et al. "Beta-adrenergic blocking drugs in the treatment of hypertension." Blood pressure vol. 10,5-6 (2001).
80. American Heart Association. "What is high blood pressure?" American Heart Association, Inc. a 501(c)(3), 2020.
81. American Heart Association. "Hypertensive crisis: When you should call 9-1-1 for high blood pressure." American Heart Association, Inc. a 501(c)(3), 2017
82. McCorry. "Physiology of the Autonomic Nervous System." The American Journal of Pharmaceutical Education, 71(4), 78, 2007.
83. Lebre. "Stress and Weight Management - Learn About the Body's Physiological Responses to Stress and Effect Stress Has on Weight Management." Today's Dietitian, 18(4), 42, 2016.
84. Delong & Sharma. "Physiology, Peripheral Vascular Resistance." StatPearls Publishing; 2019.
85. Diaz & Shimbo. "Physical activity and the prevention of hypertension." Current Hypertension Reports, 15(6), 659-668, 2014.
86. Hegde & Solomon. "Influence of physical activity on hypertension and cardiac structure and function." Current Hypertension Reports, 17(10), 77, 2016.
87. Husain, Kazim et al. "Alcohol-induced hypertension: Mechanism and prevention." World journal of cardiology vol. 6,5, 2014.
88. "American Heart Association, Does smoking increase your high blood pressure risk?" www.heart.org/en/health-topics/high-blood-pressure/changes-you-can-make-to-manage-high-blood-pressure/smoking-high-blood-pressure-and-your-health.
89. "American Heart Association, Staying hydrated." www.heart.org/en/healthy-living/fitness/fitness-basics/staying-hydrated-staying-healthy.
90. Robiou-du-Pont, Anand et al. " Parental and offspring contribution of genetic markers of adult blood pressure in early life: The FAMILY study." Journal Pone 0186218, 2017.
91. "National Institutes of Health, High blood pressure." www.nhlbi.nih.gov/health-topics/high-blood-pressure.
92. Oparil, Zaman et al. "Pathogenesis of Hypertension" Annals of Internal Medicine Nov 4, 2003.
93. Centers for Disease Control and Prevention. "Hypertension Cascade: Hypertension Prevalence, Treatment and Control Estimates Among US Adults Aged 18 Years and Older Applying the Criteria From the American College of Cardiology and American Heart Association's 2017 Hypertension Guideline 2013–2016." US Department of Health and Human Services, 2019.

94. Siri-Tarino, Patty W et al. "Saturated fatty acids and risk of coronary heart disease: modulation by replacement nutrients." Current atherosclerosis reports vol. 12,6 (2010).

95. Katan, M B et al. "Trans fatty acids and their effects on lipoproteins in humans." Annual review of nutrition vol. 15, 1995.

96. Riccardi, G et al. "Dietary fat, insulin sensitivity and the metabolic syndrome." Clinical nutrition (Edinburgh, Scotland) vol. 23,4 (2004).

97. Rivellese, Angela A et al. "Type of dietary fat and insulin resistance." Annals of the New York Academy of Sciences vol. 967 (2002).

98. Fernandez, Maria Luz. "Effects of eggs on plasma lipoproteins in healthy populations." Food & function vol. 1,2 (2010).

99. Radzevičienė, Lina, and Rytas Ostrauskas. "Egg consumption and the risk of type 2 diabetes mellitus: a case-control study." Public health nutrition vol. 15,8 (2012).

100. Pearce, Karma L et al. "Egg consumption as part of an energy-restricted high-protein diet improves blood lipid and blood glucose profiles in individuals with type 2 diabetes." The British journal of nutrition vol. 105,4 (2011).

101. "Centers for Disease Control and Prevention, Role of Sodium in Your Food." https://www.cdc.gov/salt/role_of_sodium.htm.

102. U.S. Food and Drug Administration. "Code of Federal Regulations, Title 21, Volume 2, Chapter 1, Subchapter B, Part 101 Food Labeling, Subpart D, Section 101.61 Nutrient content claims for the sodium content of foods." 2020.

103. U.S. Department of Agriculture. "Dietary Guidelines for Americans Ninth Edition." USDA Publication #: USDA-FNS-2020-2025-DGA, 2020.

104. McDonald. "The Protein Book: A Complete Guide for the Athlete and Coach." Lyle McDonald Publishing, 2007.

105. ServSafe National Restaurant Association. "ServSafe Manager, 6e." National Restaurant Association Educational Foundation, 2014.

106. "United States Department of Agriculture, Safe minimum internal temperature chart." www.fsis.usda.gov/safetempchart.

107. "UDSA Food Safety and Inspection Service, Food Handling & Preparation." www.fsis.usda.gov/food-safety.

Made in the USA
Las Vegas, NV
15 January 2023

65635592R00122